Tummy Tied

AN EASY TO DIGEST GUIDE
FOR THOSE SUFFERING WITH IBS.

By Scarlett Dixon

(KNOWN ONLINE AS *Scarlett London*)

www.iamselfpublishing.com

Disclaimer

Every effort has been made to ensure that the information in this book is
accurate at the time of publishing. The author cannot accept any responsibil-
ity for the misuse or misunderstanding of any of the information contained
herein, or any damage, loss or injury, whether its health, wellbeing, financial
or otherwise, suffered by any individual or group acting on or relying upon the
information contained within this book. The opinions contained in this book
are not intended to replace medical opinion or professional advice. If you have
any concerns about your health, please seek professional help. This has been
prepared for general information only and medical advice should be sought.

Contents

Foreword

If you're reading this, then I am possibly the happiest girl in the world right now because it means that my lifelong dream of writing a book has come true.

Given, it's not quite the fiction novel, using superlative words to describe a magical new world inspired by J.K. Rowling, that I originally had in mind, but who knows, maybe that will come in the future.

But it is a book, with an intended reader and a purpose behind it. And that's definitely good enough for me.

Before we get started, I want to thank my wonderful family for the unconditional love and support they have given me over the years – without them, I would be very lost.

Regardless of the period in my life that I was going through and how much or how little IBS affected me at that time, they have always believed in me and inspired me to go after my dreams, however farfetched they may have initially seemed.

They've always instilled in me a quietly confident mindset, and for that, I can only say thank you and I love you.

I also want to thank my boyfriend, who has aided my recovery and always provided me with love, support and reassurance – even though he himself might not have had experience of IBS personally.

He always tries to see things from my point of view and lovingly assures me that there's nothing to be embarrassed about, even if tummy turmoil is a SLIGHT intimacy killer in some instances.

Through his enduring support, and that of my family, I have learned not punish my mind and body for putting me through hideous IBS symptoms. And to accept and love myself for everything that I am. However ridiculously cliche that might sound.

Instead, I cut myself some slack and try to see the positive in every given situation.

For some (and for me in the past) IBS may be a curse, but I now truly see it as a blessing in disguise.

And here's why…

My Background

If you've picked up this book, then the chances are you are interested in finding out a little more about IBS, or *Irritable Bowel Syndrome* as it's perhaps less sympathetically called.

Whether you have the condition yourself, or a loved one has just been diagnosed, this book aims to shed a little more light into what it can be like living with dysfunctional digestive disorder (I promise I'll stop calling it all the hideously unsympathetic names under the sun) and how I've put a stop to it ruling my life.

In a nutshell, IBS is a chronic digestive condition whose symptoms are characterised by bloating, abdominal pain, excessive gas, diarrhoea and constipation. For many people, these symptoms can occur on a daily basis.

One in five people in the Western World suffers from IBS. So it affects millions of us, some more severely, while for others, it's a minor inconvenience.

And while doctors' diagnosis of the condition is on the rise, there are unfortunately only limited statistics on any kind of 'solution' to the problem.

As a brief disclaimer, I am not, by any means, a GP, Medical Professional, Nutritionist or expert, but I am an IBS sufferer who has come through the other side of the hideous symptoms and hope to impart some of my experience, knowledge and 'tummy taming' wisdom to you.

I'll also recount some of my rather embarrassing IBS related tales, so that you can rest assured that you're not alone with your tummy turmoil.

I speak to several different coaches, therapists and health practitioners who have some advice for me, as we sit down for a Q&A session together.

And I'll also share the stories of some of my fellow sufferers, who also have a couple of additional pearls of IBS-related wisdom for you.

I have been bedbound by my IBS in the past, so much so that I thought, at one point, it would truly be the end of me, my hopes, my dreams and my love life.

The symptoms can be totally unforgiving, unrelenting and all-consuming; however, as it's an invisible illness - to people on the outside, a sufferer can look totally normal and put together.

So it's frustratingly difficult to illustrate to a non-sufferer quite how much it can affect an individual's everyday life.

This is my own personal experience, so perhaps not all of the topics will be relevant to you, but having spoken to thousands of you online already, I know that some of my suggestions have helped. I do hope this book can provide further guidance, reassurance and a virtual friend to those of you who may be battling with digestive symptoms on a day-to-day basis, or have a friend, family member or partner who has recently been diagnosed with IBS or a related digestive disorder.

Both audience types are equally as important to me because it is often the support of those around you who can make a huge difference to the recovery process.

IBS can be a very isolating, confusing and debilitating condition to try and understand, and much of the advice that is already available to us online falls into one of two categories.

The first of which is very formal, medical-expert advice, featuring lots of intimidating clinical jargon, which tends to suggest there are several 'set-in-stone steps' you must take to rid yourself of the symptoms.

It doesn't delve into emotional and mental wellbeing, nor does it usually provide contextual, empathetic advice for someone suffering from the condition.

It can occasionally, and unintentionally, trivialise IBS by emphasising that it is a non-serious condition. This can isolate sufferers even further as they become concerned whether or not they should 'not cause such a fuss' or 'make a mountain out of a molehill' as it's seemingly so common.

The latter online advice resides in faceless, nameless forums, which can start to look rather 'doom and gloom' as you unravel pages upon pages of stories, conflicting advice and promotions of various different products.

Neither options are very helpful when you're trying to figure out where on earth to start with the mind-boggling condition that is IBS.

It's a minefield.

This book aims to be your go-to guide for all things IBS. A light-hearted cross between a memoir and a self- help guide.

We'll have a cry, perhaps a laugh or two and, hopefully, at the end, you'll finish with a reignited sense of 'I CAN do this'.

Again, as a disclaimer – I am not an expert by any means. I am not a qualified nutritionist and I am certainly not a doctor. *Sorry mum!* But I am an IBS sufferer. I've been through it myself. I know what boat you're in. In fact, I'm very much in the same boat.

Hopefully, this said boat has a decent toilet, eh?

IBS tends to take control of a sufferer's life, and this can be extremely unforgiving and upsetting.

This book will guide you through the process of taking back that control once and for all.

And hopefully, it will also reassure you that you're not alone.

And that you don't have to suffer in silence any longer.

No one needs to feel tongue-tied when it comes to talking about their struggles.

Or should I say, *Tummy Tied?*

I want this book to be the guide and reassurance that could have helped me at the age of 14 when I was sad, isolated and embarrassed by the new 'IBS' label that had been unwittingly placed upon me. The book I never had but that I would have loved to read.

Just to set the scene of who I am, because let's face it, we're about to delve into the realms of TMI (aka 'too much information') anyway, so I may as well introduce myself properly first.

My name is Scarlett Dixon – although I'm known on the internet as 'Scarlett London'.

My first ever memory of a 'tummy turmoil' incident was on my eighth birthday when I was sent home from school. I vividly remember being in so much pain with my stomach that the teacher discovered me curled up in a ball in the corner of the classroom.

My mum picked me up, took me home and I was on the toilet for about two hours.

As far back as I can recall, I've had a 'sensitive' tummy.

I also remember being on a surfing trip with my family in Cornwall aged 11 and having a painful urge to go to the toilet WHILE I was diving through the waves on a board. I won't tell you whether or not I made it because the story isn't my finest and we've only just met.

Indeed, my stomach and it's various quirks have always been an integral (and memorable) part of my life.

We'll talk more about that later.

I started my blog in 2011 (scarlettlondon.com) when the internet was a very different looking digital landscape. Being a 'blogger' wasn't a career choice back then, it was something you simply did as a hobby, a means of sharing your life (or in my case, passions) online. I'm pretty sure that for the first year, my only loyal reader was my mum.

I then trained as a journalist at Bournemouth University and in 2016 was awarded a First Class Honours degree in Multi-Media Journalism. Graduating was the single proudest moment in my life so far, partly because I'd worked so blooming hard and also because at several points during those three turbulent years of studying, I was so poorly with IBS I thought I'd have to quit.

I left university and started working in lifestyle and fashion journalism, spending time at a number of women's magazines in the UK. I was working in London, commuting daily and trying to balance kick-starting my career and running my blog.

In 2017, I decided to go 'full time' with my blog – a nerve-wracking decision, but also a very exciting one, since I was able to have full control over my working schedule and build a business that was totally my own. It also meant that I didn't have to answer to anyone with regards to managing my symptoms, nor did I have to feel guilty when I was too poorly to go into an office.

It also meant that I had a lot more free time (i.e. the two hours I didn't have to spend commuting) to research what IBS really entailed and in turn to discover how I could finally take back control of my life, and get rid of the hideous symptoms I'd been suffering with for so long.

My business is now in its second year of trading and my day-to-day is very varied. I'm genuinely excited and enthused about everything I do. I work with global brands on partnerships and campaigns, I organise large-scale networking events for 'social media influencers' and content creators and I run my social channels to produce content that hopefully brings a daily dose of positivity to someone's newsfeed.

It's a bit of light-hearted relief from the constant stream of online vitriol and overwhelmingly negative news stories.

My lifelong dream is to become an author and write books for a living. I suppose you could say I'm getting there!

Back in the early days of blogging, I started out with a platform to share my views on the 'lipstick of the moment' or provide a snapshot of my 'outfit of the day'. It wasn't until much later that I began opening up, sharing more of my personal life and using it as a therapeutic outlet to write about my worries, fears and aspirations.

The pinnacle moment occurred in 2013, as while hundreds of miles away from home at university, my relationship of four years ended, and my IBS reared its ugly head for the umpteenth time.

I hadn't made any friends yet (because it was only my second week) and I didn't have anyone to talk to, so having previously kept my IBS struggles a secret from all but my mum, I decided, for whatever reason, to pour my heart into a blog post, revealing what I'd been suffering from for so long.

And finding my voice was scary, but exactly what I needed.

I expected a few people to turn their noses up, a couple to relate and perhaps – at a push – for it to help at least ONE person.

But the reaction I received blew me away. To this day, I still receive between five and 30 emails a week from sufferers all around the world, who bravely share their own IBS story with me over the internet.

This is very much part of the reason I wanted to put this book together – because the emails, messages and comments I receive on a daily basis are wonderful, but I don't always have the time to reply to them in the depth I would like. I want to reassure everyone that they're not alone. And they don't have to be solitary in navigating this crazy, frustrating and isolating condition.

The book will be divided into separate topics that I think each deserve their own space and their own chapter. They will sound out issues that affect that particular subject and provide coping mechanisms that I (or the case studies) suggest might be helpful for you to try. In each section, I share anecdotes about my life - ranging from the frustrating, to the upsetting, to the downright mortifying – but they're potentially pretty funny. You'll also find Q&A's with some wonderful people in my life who have supported me - as well as tips and tricks that you can easily implement in your daily life.

The aim of the game is for you to come away feeling less alone, more equipped with the tools (physical and mental) to deal with your IBS symptoms and to encourage you to join the movement of talking about digestive health.

Through sharing my story online, I have created something of a community. This has been the most rewarding thing for me to see, because for so long, I thought that I was the only person who existed with IBS symptoms like mine.

So don't be shy, speak up, and if you see another person reading this book on the train, in the airport, on the beach or in your workplace, go and say hello. If you snap a picture together - tag me and I'll share it on my social media too! I'm over at @scarlettlondon on Instagram

By doing so, together, we will ensure that IBS doesn't have to be a taboo subject.

And that no-one has to suffer in silence.

Or be *Tummy Tied*.

The Poo Taboo

One in five people in the UK have been diagnosed with IBS. Apparently, it's slightly more common in women than in men (perhaps to do with the fact that us women have a longer colon than men and hormones can affect our digestion), but that's essentially 20% of the population. A figure I found ASTONISHING.

And yet despite this, little is known about the condition itself. The causes are unknown and any official research over the past decade has been fairly minimal.

When researching for a university project back in 2015, I discovered the NHS spends over £400 million every year on prescribing IBS-related medicines, although I imagine that figure has risen year on year.

For all those that have been 'officially' diagnosed, there are also many silent sufferers, who haven't visited the doctors about their symptoms or suffer a mild form and are content with self-treating.

IBS isn't picky, it affects people in all different situations in their lives, in varying job roles, including people of different ages and races.

Essentially, IBS is an umbrella term for a collection of symptoms that all relate to digestive dysfunction. It is a chronic condition and, at present, there is no one size fits all cure. I'll be going into depth further in the book about the methods I have used to treat and improve my IBS symptoms but before we get started, I thought that it would be helpful to talk a little bit about each of those individual symptoms, so that you can identify which of them you are finding most difficult to deal with.

Symptoms can differ in severity from person to person and an IBS sufferer may not get ALL of the textbook symptoms at once. Certain digestive issues may fluctuate or come and go.

Often it's a little overwhelming to try and target ALL of the symptoms at once. And you may find different digestive issues react to different treatment methods. For example, the bloating I have targeted via my diet, whereas the low mood and hormonal flare-ups I have targeted through CBT, coaching and medication.

In this chapter, I'll talk a little bit about treatment methods and tips I've found helpful to try and deal with each symptom individually, but I will also go into greater depth as we move through the book – so don't be disappointed if

I skip over certain subjects. There's more to come, don't you worry!

As with ANY new or persistent symptom, you should always visit your doctor to rule out any underlying conditions before self-diagnosing. It's important to figure out whether your symptoms are as a result of IBS or whether they are caused by something else entirely. Typically, doctors in the UK like to monitor your potential IBS symptoms for a period of three months or more; suggesting keeping a food diary and conducting blood tests to rule out Crohn's, UC (Ulcerative Colitis), IBD (Irritable Bowel Disease) or Coeliac. The latter of which has similar symptoms but can be life-threatening in rare cases, so I cannot stress the importance of seeking professional medical advice enough.

This is by no means an exhaustive list of symptoms, it is just those that I have personally experienced and those I know so many of you also suffer most from.

From the outset, and when experienced in acute bouts, some of the issues can seem pretty trivial to the outsider.

However, for the person suffering, they really can be hideously debilitating and affect daily life - especially when they are combined together with other symptoms.

So let's get started…

CHAPTER 1

The Symptoms

DIARRHOEA

- ABDOMINAL CRAMPS
- ABDOMINAL PAINS
- URGENCY TO GO TO THE TOILET
- FREQUENT PASSING OF LOOSE, WATERY FAECES

As an IBS sufferer, you may be more prone to IBS-D (the D standing for the oh-so-fabulous diarrhoea) or IBS-C (see below) or a combination of the two. As luck would have it, I've had a real mix of each, alternating frequently.

During the second year of my university, I suffered from chronic, persistent and unrelenting diarrhoea.

Imagine having food poisoning or the stomach flu – only every single day, with no single direct cause or tummy equilibrium on the near horizon.

It's incredibly debilitating and after a short while, your entire day starts to revolve around when your bowels decide they want to unleash themselves on whatever toilet you can locate the quickest.

You feel out of control of your body and even the smallest of tasks, such as driving to work, taking the train, walking to the bus stop, standing in a queue or meeting friends in the park, turns into a huge, scary and tricky ordeal. This is because you begin to plan your days depending on where the nearest toilet is, which isn't any fun.

And more often than not, finding a toilet that you can use while you're out and about is difficult to come by, so you shelve engaging in certain activities because you don't want to be caught short.

I knew I'd hit rock bottom (excuse the pun) when I couldn't leave my bedroom (or should I say bathroom) at all because I was having to go to the toilet twelve times each morning – with a desperate and persistent urge to go again. I felt totally empty; my body wasn't absorbing any nutrients, essential vitamins and minerals from my food because it was going straight through me. I was exhausted, fed up and in tears most days. My tummy was sore and the 'urge' to go was waking me up in the night.

I was terrified to eat anything other than plain bread, rice or chicken because my stomach was so sensitive and reacted to anything I put inside it. And I felt a prisoner of my guts.

The loose stools can be either quite minor (just a little more watery than usual) or major – and it can vary depending on your stress levels, food and exercise. I have always found my sensitive stomach is irritated by the slightest of worries and so I have a series of 'butterfly belly poos' whenever I am a little nervous about something, which tends to clear out my system temporarily and then cause constipation.

What helped me with this symptom?

- A PROBIOTIC DAILY HELPED TO SLOW THINGS DOWN AND HARMONISE MY DIGESTIVE SYSTEM, SOOTHING IT AND CALMING IT

- PEPPERMINT TEA OR SUPPLEMENTS CAN ACT AS AN ANTI-SPASMODIC AND SLOW DOWN THE CONTRACTIONS OF YOUR DIGESTIVE SYSTEM, CALMING IT BACK INTO A REGULAR RHYTHM

- EATING PLAIN FOODS AND SMALL PORTIONS (MAYBE 6 SMALL MEALS A DAY)

- GETTING INTO A 'ROUTINE' WITH MY BODY ON A DAILY BASIS (BREAKFAST, TEA, POO).

- MAKING SURE I EMPTIED MYSELF PROPERLY. OFTEN WE'RE IN SUCH A RUSH IN OUR LIVES, WE DON'T ALLOW OURSELVES THE NECESSARY TIME TO ENSURE IT'S ALL 'OUT'

- CBT AND THERAPY FOR ANXIETY. I FOUND MY DIARRHOEA WAS INTENSELY CONNECTED TO ANXIETY. WHENEVER I AM ANXIOUS, I GENERALLY GO TO THE TOILET MORE OFTEN. AND WORRYING ABOUT HAVING TO GO TO THE TOILET MORE WILL, IN TURN, MAKE ME GO TO THE TOILET MORE

- PREPARING FOR EVERY EVENTUALITY WITH AN EMERGENCY STASH OF SUPPLEMENTS, MEDICATION AND WET WIPES, WHICH I CARRY ON MY PERSON AT ALL TIMES

CONSTIPATION

- PASSING FEWER THAN THREE STOOLS A WEEK (OR FEWER THAN IS NORMAL FOR YOU)

- HAVING LUMPY OR HARD STOOLS

- STRAINING TO HAVE BOWEL MOVEMENTS

- FEELING AS THOUGH THERE'S A BLOCKAGE IN YOUR RECTUM THAT PREVENTS BOWEL MOVEMENTS

- FEELING AS THOUGH YOU CAN'T COMPLETELY EMPTY THE STOOL FROM YOUR RECTUM

The other end of the spectrum, of course, is being constipated, which isn't much fun either. At my worst, I didn't 'go' for almost two weeks, by which point I was ready to burst. I was hideously uncomfortable and couldn't function properly because I felt so 'full'.

Constipation can vary from not going at all, to being able to go but not feeling completely empty after you visit the loo. The latter can be particularly frustrating because you never quite get that feeling of your bowels having completely flushed themselves out. You know that instant 'relief' after you go to the toilet? When you're constipated, that feeling is few and far between.

And it can also result in something wonderfully exciting called 'impaction', which I was diagnosed with several times throughout my 10+ years of IBS adventures – and it's fun, fun, FUN! Essentially, it means your poo is lodged inside your colon, often caused by a hard mass that gets 'stuck' and then causes an orderly queue of other poos.

At this exact moment of writing, I am currently questioning what on EARTH I am doing composing a book that shares quite THIS much detail and I sincerely apologise if you are eating or currently pondering what to have for dinner and now have been put off completely. But you know, all in the name of breaking the poo taboo, eh?

I'll never forget a skiing trip I took with a previous boy-friend many moons ago.

I was having an extreme bout of constipation at the time and hadn't gone for a couple of days before leaving. For the entire week I was away, I couldn't enjoy or focus on the task in hand because I felt so 'bogged' down by constipation, which was worrying as skiing on a blooming great mountain requires a lot of focus and attention.

I actually remember going to sleep DREAMING about having a poo because there was nothing I wanted more than to feel 'empty' and get rid of all the waste in my system. I didn't go for almost two weeks and the constant strain-ing when trying meant that I was treated to my first royal welcome from my lovely friend Mr Piles. Just some friendly advice. DO NOT GOOGLE 'piles' and then accidentally click on the images tab. Don't say I didn't warn you.

What helped me with this symptom?

- GENTLE EXERCISE AND STAYING HYDRATED

- ENSURING I HAD ENOUGH FIBRE IN MY DIET (5 FRUIT AND VEG PORTIONS PER DAY AT LEAST)

- GETTING MY BODY INTO A ROUTINE AND HAVING A BREAKFAST HIGH IN FIBRE, SUCH AS PORRIDGE, OATS, FRUIT ETC.

- TAKING A DAILY PROBIOTIC AND ADDED FIBRE SUPPLEMENTS WHENEVER NEEDED (I.E. WHEN TRAVELLING WHEN CONSTIPATION CAN OCCUR)

- MINIMISING TRIGGER FOODS THAT CAUSED CONSTIPATION SPECIFICALLY (FOR ME, TOO MANY EGGS)

BLOATING

- O A SWOLLEN STATE CAUSED BY RETENTION OF FLUID OR GAS

- O FEELING FULL, TIGHT, OR SWOLLEN IN THE ABDOMEN

- O DISTENDED, HARD, AND PAINFUL ABDOMEN

"Oh, I'm so bloated too, I just ate that HUGE pizza."

For some people, bloating is an occasional and minor inconvenience. It's the slightly uncomfortable feeling after a heavy meal, where you might need to loosen your belt or unbutton your jeans and stretch out or go for a walk. However, IBS sufferers can experience a severe form of bloating, which happens as soon as they start eating or drinking in the day, and of course, this can be incredibly uncomfortable and debilitating - eventually impeding upon daily life.

Several years ago, I suffered so severely from extreme bloating that I had to alter my entire wardrobe. If I wanted a new pair of jeans, I'd have to come to terms with the fact that I'd need to stock up on a bigger size – solely to accommodate the bloat. In fact, my clothes ranged from a size 10 to a size 16. And at university, I'd more than likely go for a bigger size or risk my clothes being too tight around my tummy, which would cause me a hideous amount of pain and discomfort.

At one point, I resigned myself to the fact that I'd never be able to choose clothes just because I actually LIKED them. Instead, the deciding factor was because they were loose around the tummy area or had a stretchy or adjustable waistband. At the time, I felt humiliated and like an old lady, however I now fully appreciate my vast collection of stretchy waistband garments, because I LOVE food and if my clothes can help me conceal my *dairy-free* pizza baby bump, then I am ALL for it.

At my worst, I was mistaken for being a couple of months pregnant. And although I didn't take it personally, (although I could have - I'd now advise people to avoid asking someone if they are pregnant UNTIL they announce it themselves – it just isn't worth the risk), it did upset me that I couldn't wear the crop top and denim jean combos that my peers at university would rock up in.

Even now, I know I'm the kind of person that would NEVER be able to wear something super tight or restrictive, purely because of the immense amount of pain it would cause me to have something really tight around my stomach. If a bloating attack did present itself, I would be in extraordinary amounts of pain.

For me, the bloating feels like someone has stuffed a basketball into my intestines and is quickly pumping it up so that it's round and uncomfortable. I wish I could say that I sported a rock solid stomach due to abs, but alas, I'll usually be rocking a hard, tight bloat. Oh so fab-u-lous!

When bloated, my stomach is full, heavy and swollen, and I feel completely uncomfortable and not-quite-myself. As my job involves taking part in photo-shoots for brands, being able to fit into a certain size of clothing or looking 'my best', it can be a difficult symptom to deal with. However, I do now have a lot more control over the bloating side of things and can pre-empt a meal that could cause me issues.

It can be a very disruptive symptom because it is so all-consuming. You feel extremely uncomfortable and may be in lots of pain with accompanying sharp, tight cramping. I tend to find that any bloating that I suffer from is partnered by a stabbing pain in the lower right side of my abdomen, as well as a tight sensation under my ribs.

What helped me with this symptom?

- FINDING THE TRIGGER FOODS THAT EXACERBATED MY BLOATING AND EITHER ELIMINATING OR MINIMISING THEM

- NOT ALWAYS EATING MY FOOD IN SUCH A RUSH AND CONSUMING FOOD MORE MINDFULLY

- HAVING A GO-TO COMFORTABLE BUT SMART OUTFIT FOR OCCASIONS WHEN I WANTED TO FEEL GOOD, BUT DID NOT WANT TO RESTRICT A BLOATED BELLY

- HOT WATER BOTTLE, HEAT COMPRESSIONS AND PEPPERMINT TEA ON STANDBY

- STRETCHING OUT YOUR STOMACH AND KEEPING ACTIVE THROUGHOUT THE DAY – TRY NOT TO BE HUNCHED IN A CERTAIN POSITION ALL DAY LONG

- MASSAGING MY ABDOMEN AREA GENTLY

ABDOMINAL PAIN

- CRAMPING

- TUMMY ACHE

- STABBING OR SHOOTING PAINS

- TENDER AND SWOLLEN ABDOMEN

- CONSTANT DULL ACHE IN THE STOMACH

Back in the days when I was too afraid to actually tell anyone what I was suffering from, I'd downplay my various symptoms as 'stomach ache'. It seemed easier for people to understand that way, plus I didn't have to go into any embarrassing detail and individuals didn't ask too many questions as a follow-up.

A bit of tummy ache is pretty common here and there, but the abdominal pain that is often described by IBS sufferers can be a mixture of intense cramping, stabbing pains, a 'full sensation', a sore and tender stomach, or a general uneasy nauseous and dull stomach ache.

It can also be used to describe the sensation of getting an 'urge' to go to the toilet. This can often be immediate, painful and uncomfortable, and may not subside after actually visiting the bathroom. I used to joke to my mum that my stomach was in a constant state of pain; this just varied in intensity, depending on the time of day. And, unfortunately, I know this is also true for so many of you too.

As with any chronic pain, it can be incredibly debilitating and difficult to figure out. I felt fed up and frustrated that my body couldn't tell me what it needed to fix this particular pain, nor could I seem to figure out what caused it.

I'll talk about this in far more depth later on in the book, but I later discovered that a huge contributor of pain for me was caused by eating dairy. My body lacks the enzymes needed to digest both the lactose AND the proteins found in dairy, so after consumption, it would sit in my large intestine, ferment and cause me an immense amount of pain, discomfort and cramping.

I do still suffer from abdominal pain occasionally, but I choose to 'punish myself less' and try not to get so frustrated about it. Abdominal pain was probably the symptom I felt angry about most because it cast a huge shadow over my life and didn't allow me to get on with my day-to-day activities like everyone else. I always had this nagging stomach ache, which would cause anxiety and worry, so getting myself out of this downward cycle was key.

What helped me with this symptom?

- CUTTING OUT DAIRY AND PINPOINTING TRIGGER FOODS (I'D SAY THIS REDUCED THE SEVERITY OF THIS SYMPTOM BY 85-90%)

- HOT WATER BOTTLES AND HEAT COMPRESSIONS

- PEPPERMINT OR FRESH MINT TEA

- A DAILY PROBIOTIC

- DIGESTIVE ENZYME SUPPLEMENTS

- BEING KINDER TO MYSELF (GETTING FRUSTRATED ONLY EXACERBATED THE PAIN)

EXCESSIVE & TRAPPED WIND

- PASSING EXCESSIVE GAS FROM THE DIGESTIVE SYSTEM OUT OF THE BACK PASSAGE

- EXCESSIVE FLATULENCE CAN BE EMBARRASSING AND MAKE YOU FEEL UNCOMFORTABLE AROUND OTHERS

- A BUILD-UP OF GAS IN THE DIGESTIVE SYSTEM, WHICH CAN CAUSE PAIN AND DISCOMFORT

Gas, wind, farting, trumping or 'popping off' as my sister calls it (a term which makes me laugh every time I hear it) – they are all names for the same pretty normal bodily function. According to many health websites, it's perfectly normal to fart and, on average, people do it between 5 and 15 times a day. I can't say I've ever counted or tracked my farts on a daily basis, but I'm pretty sure that during my worst flare-ups, my number would be double or even triple that. It's clearly one thing I exceed expectations on.

Gas can often become trapped in the digestive system, causing shooting pains, cramping and a build-up of toxins.

Trapped wind tends to be caused by bacteria in the colon working overtime and producing excessive amounts of gas bubbles which can be difficult to pass. This can then be exacerbated if you hold in the said gas because it produces a build-up and a distended abdomen (aka bloating, as above).

Obviously, we can't always let out gas all of the time. It's seen as impolite if you're in public or in company, which is why many of us get into a cycle of holding in gas. This, in turn, can cause further bouts of trapped wind.

Excessive wind and trapped wind can both be extremely debilitating because they become quite all-consuming and uncomfortable, especially if you are around others on a daily basis – either at work or in social situations.

What helped me with this symptom?

- ELIMINATING TRIGGER FOODS – DAIRY CAUSED A LOT OF WIND FOR ME, AS DOES ONION OCCASIONALLY

- LETTING IT OUT, WHENEVER POSSIBLE – HOLDING IT IN ONLY CAUSES MORE PAIN (GO FOR A 10 MINUTE WALK AROUND THE BLOCK IF YOU NEED TO GET OUT OF THE OFFICE)

- HAVING A DAILY PROBIOTIC

- STRETCHING AND DOING GENTLE EXERCISE

- NOT EATING TOO MUCH REFINED SUGAR (I STICK TO MAPLE SYRUP IF I NEED SOMETHING SWEET TO ADD TO MY FOOD)

MUCUS

Before I started researching IBS symptoms, I had no idea that passing mucus when you go to the toilet is actually very normal. In order for your colon to move all your waste product through your bowel, a mucus lining is present to protect the inner layer of our digestive system.

Mucus is an important fluid produced by our bodies to protect our nose, throat, lungs and sinuses from infection. So in a way, it's a good thing to see it. It means your body is working and protecting itself.

However, if you notice an increased amount when you are going to the toilet, or you are JUST passing mucus rather than anything else (which is something I get quite a lot), then it's worth consulting your doctor about it.

This applies to any changes you might notice when you go to the toilet, such as blood, mucus etc. In fact, several years ago, when I was at my very worst, I passed a large amount of blood and mucus when I went to the toilet and it was scary. Terrifying. Largely because it's not something you feel you can appropriately chat about to other people (so you're not sure if it's normal) and also because it's sometimes a cause for concern and is definitely something you should get checked out for. Peace of mind and reassurance can actually HELP your symptoms, especially if, like me, you create more anxiety and worry by thinking about what those symptoms mean, which in turn, causes a flare-up.

More often than not, mucus can be a sign of inflammation (I always get it when I eat something my body doesn't agree with, like gelatine) and fresh blood can be a sign of straining too hard. But it's always worth getting it checked out for total peace of mind and the best chance of managing your symptoms as effectively as possible.

What helped me with this symptom?

- NOT EATING TRIGGER FOODS – FOR WHATEVER REASON, I FIND THAT EATING JELLY AND GELATINE CAUSES MORE MUCUS

- ENSURING I EAT ENOUGH FIBRE

- ENSURING I EAT A HEALTHY, BALANCED AND NUTRITIOUS DIET THAT GIVES MY BODY ALL THE RIGHT NUTRIENTS IT NEEDS

- STAYING HYDRATED

FOOD INTOLERANCES

- DIFFICULTY DIGESTING CERTAIN FOODS

- HAVING AN UNPLEASANT PHYSICAL REACTION TO CERTAIN FOODS

- BLOATING AND STOMACH PAINS AFTER EATING CERTAIN FOODS

- SKIN RASHES AND ITCHING AFTER CERTAIN FOODS

Food intolerances occur when your gut is very sensitive and reacts to certain foods that may trigger the production of excess gas, cramping or bloating. Most people with IBS or digestive complaints will have certain food intolerances, even if they are not immediately evident.

For some people, a food intolerance upset might occur after they have eaten too much of a certain food (they may be able to tolerate a little bit of it) and more severe food intolerances may be flared up by even a small amount. It varies from person to person and we will go into more depth about food intolerances and the role that the identification of 'trigger' foods can play in improving your IBS and obtaining more control over your symptoms.

For me, I can react quite severely to certain foods, so much so that I have to totally avoid them. In the past, I found this really limiting and difficult, but I now consider it one of my 'quirks' and use it as a means of encouraging me to live a healthy and balanced lifestyle.

However, that's not to say that I haven't found it troublesome in the past, especially in social situations, as it can feel quite daunting having to present your host (or a waitress) with a long list of items you can't have. I've been called fussy, difficult, strange and restrictive by both friends and strangers. It wasn't until I had to give up certain foods to manage my symptoms that I realised just how much of our social lives revolve around food. In fact, how much of our lives, in general revolve, around food.

There are certain foods I love that, unfortunately, don't love me back and it's certainly been a bit of a tug of war between 'do I want to feel well?' and 'do I want to eat something delicious?'. But I have learned to appreciate the feeling of when food DOES love my body back.

What helped me with this symptom?

- GETTING TESTED PRIVATELY FOR ALLERGIES

- KEEPING A FOOD DIARY

- ELIMINATING TRIGGER FOODS

HORMONAL FLARE-UPS

- O AN INCREASE IN SYMPTOMS AROUND YOUR
     MONTHLY CYCLE

- O AN INCREASE IN THE SEVERITY OF YOUR
     IBS SYMPTOMS AROUND THE TIME OF YOUR
     MONTHLY PERIOD OR OVULATION

Obviously this particular symptom is only relevant to those who menstruate (so feel free to skip this if you don't) however up until very recently, I didn't fully appreciate how intricately connected our hormones are to our guts. It was only when I downloaded a period tracking app about a year ago that allowed me to input mood, bowel changes and bloating that I started to notice a pattern emerge.

About a week before I was due to start my period, I noticed an increase in the number of toilet trips I was having, and then once my period arrived, I went completely the other way and was constipated for a few days until the end of my bleeding cycle.

After further research into this topic, I noted that the sex hormones "oestrogen" and "progesterone", which play an important role in controlling a woman's menstrual cycle, have 'receptor cells' located inside the digestive tract. So it makes perfect sense for the digestive function to be affected by the changing levels of these hormones throughout the monthly cycle, even if this occurs in just a minor way.

During a period, the sex hormones are at their lowest, so it is possible to notice an increase in the severity or appearance of your IBS symptoms.

Obviously, these hormones can be unpredictable and seemingly 'unmanageable'; however, I found a lot of relief from the effect of them on my IBS symptoms AFTER I came off the contraceptive pill last year. Having been on varying doses and brands of the pill for almost 10 years (and really not getting along very well with the mood changes, weight gain and other side effects) I decided, after careful consultation with my nurse, GP and my boyfriend, to see how coming off it would affect my symptoms.

It's going to vary for everyone because each individual has a different reaction to each medication, but for me, not having synthetic hormones in my body meant that my IBS symptoms were far less severe. Later down the line, a friend pointed out to me that the pill contains (albeit in a very very small dose) lactose and milk sugars, which IBS sufferers can be sensitive to. So this could also have also been a contributing factor in my symptoms improving.

As a disclaimer again, I am NOT a medical professional nor am I advising you to change your medication. This is purely my personal story and, of course, contraception is a very personal choice that I would never want to impinge upon. But all of these factors are worth considering in the construction of your IBS management plan, so do consult your healthcare professional if you think this could be a factor affecting your symptoms. There's also no harm in downloading the free period tracking app 'Clue', so you can log your symptoms alongside where you are in your cycle. It has a specific tracker for 'bowel movements' so you can input in each day whether you were constipated, gassy or had diarrhoea.

What helped me with this symptom?

- DOWNLOADING A PERIOD TRACKER SO I KNEW WHEN TO EXPECT HORMONAL FLARE-UPS/ COINCIDING SYMPTOMS

- KEEPING A REGULAR MORNING ROUTINE

- USING NON-HORMONAL CONTRACEPTIVE METHODS

- USING PADS INSTEAD OF TAMPONS (I FOUND TAMPONS COULD GET IN THE WAY AND MAKE ME FEEL LESS HYGIENIC IF I HAD A FLARE-UP AND WAS OUT AND ABOUT)

NEGATIVE BODY IMAGE

- O SELF-CRITICISM

- O OBSESSIVE SELF-SCRUTINY IN MIRRORS

- O DISPARAGING THOUGHTS ABOUT YOUR BODY

Another not so obvious symptom of IBS can involve having a negative body image, as a result of the severe bloating related to the condition. There have been times when I've felt so bloated that I've cried in front of the mirror at my bulging, swollen stomach. Often when I've been travelling and the foods are differ from what I'm used to back at home, my bloating can be at its worst - which means that going out and exploring my exciting new surroundings can feel very intimidating.

I remember a gorgeous candle-lit dinner on the beach one night in Thailand when I changed my outfit five times before finally feeling comfortable enough in something. It wasn't the pretty, body-con red dress I wanted to wear, but an old floaty skirt that I'd bought five years ago (and quite frankly, had seen better days). It was the only thing I could fit around my bulging, sore stomach. All night, I poked and prodded at my stomach, feeling low about the way I looked and felt. This is such a sad thought because I should have been concentrating on the wonderfully romantic night we'd planned.

I've struggled with a negative body image my whole life and can remember being on fad diets as far back as the age of 13. I frequently compared my body to Britney Spears' washboard abs, which were plastered all over the covers of magazines. My body definitely didn't match up so I punished it by cutting out meals, I scrutinised it in the mirror and obsessively looked at other women and celebrities, comparing my body to theirs. I had an unhealthy relationship with my body and saw myself as the enemy. I would pick apart the person in the mirror with intense scrutiny; something I wouldn't even dream of doing to someone I disliked. This was totally bizarre looking back but I think it was partly down to societal pressures that I was this way, perhaps exacerbated by IBS symptoms.

Now I make a conscious effort to partake in daily 'affirmations', which sounds hippy-dippy but they are actually a fantastic means of retraining HOW you look at yourself in the mirror. It becomes all too easy when we look at our reflection to let our eyes dart straight to what we deem to be the 'flaws'. But your body is fantastic, it's beautiful, unique, fabulous and incredible. It houses you, keeps you alive – and is the only place you LIVE. So we really should treat it like our temple, take good care of it and look after it with loving thoughts.

Rather than looking in the mirror and being disparaging, it has really helped me to get into a habit of being complimentary about what I see staring back at me. Daily affirmations can include 'you look beautiful', or 'I am strong'. Find one that resonates with you and then repeat it back to yourself daily for 7 days. It sounds terribly cringe-worthy and narcissistic (or perhaps we are made to think that it is), but its oh so good for the mind.

I know it's easier said than done when you've got a bloated belly staring back at you, but give it a try, make yourself laugh and have fun with it.

There's only one of you, so celebrate that!

What helped me with this symptom?

- CBT

- CREATING MY '9 RULES TO LIFE'

- WRITING DOWN MY EMOTIONS, FEELINGS AND THOUGHTS

- COMMUNICATING WITH OTHERS HOW I WAS FEELING

- INTRODUCING POSITIVE AFFIRMATIONS

LOW MOOD

- O   SADNESS

- O   FEELING ANXIOUS OR PANICKY

- O   WORRY

- O   TIREDNESS

- O   LOW SELF-ESTEEM

- O   FRUSTRATION

We'll talk more about anxiety and the emotional impact that digestive disorders can have later in the book. As I feel this is such an underreported topic, it deserves its very own chapter. One of the main reasons I wanted to put this guide together was because I felt the literature and books that are already out there give incredible practical advice, but they barely scratch the surface of the emotional toll that IBS can have on an individual. Often, it's the most difficult 'symptom' to deal with and yet it's the least spoken about. I feel the benefit of having a 'personal' story to tell (if you can call it that) is that I want to underpin this aspect to all of the advice and practical tips I provide.

At my lowest point, when I was 21, I spent every single day in tears. It was awful, hideous and I couldn't see a way out. I remember sitting on the edge of my bed, sobbing while my then-boyfriend stared at me, unaware of what to do or what to say. It must have been awful not being able to help, but I took out a lot of my frustrations on him and there was a lot of arguing and sadness, which only made me feel even more miserable. I remember once blurting out, 'I think I'm depressed' because I almost NEEDED to put a label on the rollercoaster of emotions that I was going through.

I was later put on anti-depressants and eventually signed off university by a doctor who bluntly told me that I '*had a lot of emotions to deal with*'. Quite right, I do. But I now know how to manage those emotions and not let them run away with me so that they don't cause a downward spiral. I practice CBT and mindfulness (which I'll talk about in more detail later in the book) and it helps me to think of my emotions as waves. My thoughts and feelings come and go like waves in the ocean, but it's up to me to control which ones to surf.

IBS can leave you feeling so out of control. Low mood is an obvious side effect of the other symptoms, but it's not heavily publicised, so we need to make sure that we look out for one another and hand out smiles whenever we can. You never know what the person sitting opposite you is going through, just as they don't know how you are feeling. Be kind, whenever you can. Kindness is so underrated, but can make someone's day a little bit better - so use it freely!

What helped me with this symptom?

- CBT

- ACKNOWLEDGING MY FEELINGS WERE THERE, INSTEAD OF IGNORING THEM

- PUTTING BUILDING BLOCKS IN PLACE IN CERTAIN ASPECTS OF MY LIFE TO HELP ME FEEL MORE IN CONTROL

- ORGANISING MY LIFE USING A 'CHECKLIST' JOURNAL AND HAVING DAILY TO-DO LISTS TO HELP ME FEEL PRODUCTIVE, WHILE KEEPING ME BUSY

- GENTLE EXERCISE

- ENOUGH SLEEP

- CONFIDING IN FRIENDS AND FAMILY

FATIGUE

- EXTREME/CHRONIC TIREDNESS AND SLEEPINESS

- DIZZINESS

- SORENESS OF THE MUSCLES

- SLOWED REFLEXES AND RESPONSES

- IMPAIRED DECISION MAKING AND JUDGEMENT

This aspect of IBS isn't as well documented as the more 'obvious' symptoms; however, it's something that I'm sure many people with a chronic illness can relate to – and it's certainly an issue that has affected my life quite drastically since my IBS diagnosis.

I'd always been a very energetic person (you'll hear from my mum later in the book, who has a delightful story that highlights quite how energy efficient I was in the morning), but things changed about a year after my initial IBS diagnosis.

Over the Christmas break, aged 15, I was struck down by a nasty bout of glandular fever. It totally wiped me out for several months, as the Epstein-Barr virus ravished my body. It left me with no voice for four weeks (and a throat that felt like I was swallowing razor blades) and glands so swollen my whole face was puffy and disfigured. For months, I was only well enough to go into school for either morning or afternoon sessions, and I slept for the rest of the day.

I never really made a 'full' recovery. In fact, I recently had tests which showed that the Epstein-Barr virus was still active in my system, almost 10 years after being diagnosed. Unfortunately, my IBS symptoms seemed to exacerbate my tiredness.

Throughout my GCSEs, I would attend school, come home at 3pm and sleep until 6pm, then wake up for dinner and an hour or two's revision, before going back to sleep until the morning. Some may have put it down to 'lazy teenager' syndrome, but for me, this exhaustion and chronic tiredness was a very real symptom that I struggled with. My social life practically vanished and it was hard for me to verbalise to friends quite how it was affecting me.

Fatigue is something that has been an ongoing symptom for me. This is frustrating but also motivating in the sense that it encourages me to lead an active healthy lifestyle. I sleep at least 7-8 hours a night, drink plenty of water and have a healthy balanced diet, which minimises the tiredness. If I don't achieve the desired number of hours of sleep per night, I find my IBS symptoms worsen. Quite recently, I had a rather nasty and terrifying bout of sleep paralysis as a direct result of not getting enough sleep during my travels – and my symptoms DID NOT like that at all. So I understand and appreciate my limits.

Fatigue is a very underestimated part of IBS. This is especially true if you're prone to IBS-D and your body is suffering from malabsorption or even IBS-C where you are so lethargic and exhausted from being full, bloated and swollen.

Not having the energy to complete even the most simple daily tasks can be frustrating, debilitating and difficult to deal with, especially if there's no immediate relief on the horizon.

What helped me with this symptom?

- A NUTRITIOUS DIET AND ENOUGH SLEEP EACH NIGHT

- STAYING HYDRATED

- IRON SUPPLEMENTS (I USE THE SPA-TONE LIQUID SACHETS AS I'VE FOUND THAT THEY ARE MORE GENTLE ON YOUR STOMACH THAN OTHER IRON SUPPLEMENTS)

STOMACH NOISES

- ○   ALSO KNOWN AS BORBORYGMI

- ○   REFERS TO THE STOMACH SOUNDS CREATED BY
    AIR OR FLUID MOVING AROUND THE SMALL AND
    LARGE INTESTINES.

- ○   STOMACH MUSCLES CONTRACT AND MOVE
    CONTENTS ONWARDS IN THE DIGESTIVE TRACT,
    CREATING SOUNDS A RUMBLING OR GURGLING
    NOISE THAT CAN BE VERY QUIET OR VERY LOUD

- ○   A BUBBLING SENSATION IN THE GUT WHICH CAN
    BE UNCOMFORTABLE

In an initial video that I posted on my YouTube channel, I mentioned rather fleetingly about the windy, angry alien grumbles that exploded from my stomach and it seemed to resonate with many of you, who said you have experienced the same thing.

I perhaps played down the role these ridiculous noises had on my teenage years, but they were so tough to deal with when at school, confined to a classroom, with thirty other students, while trying to focus my mind and take in what I was supposed to be learning about. Yet my stomach was wailing away, trying to attract attention and causing me to feel utterly mortified in the process.

School and your educational years are tricky enough to navigate, so you can imagine what it's like when you throw dealing with IBS into the mix.

If you're also a sufferer of the windy, angry alien grumbles, here are some other handy tips to follow:

Learn to laugh at yourself

We often feel embarrassed about our tummy noises, which makes us panic. We feel that the physical noises will 'reveal' our tummy turmoil to our peers and unveil the big secret that we've been keeping to ourselves for so long. This doesn't have to be the case, and if you're the kind of person to feel comfortable doing so, just make a joke about it. Laugh about it. This can trick the brain and stop you going into panic mode. Now if my tummy has decided to do its weird thing, I will poke it and say 'sorry about the angry alien in there' or 'excuse the tiger in my tummy today'. We forget everyone has tummy noises from time to time. They're normal and nothing to be embarrassed about. Plus everyone is SO focused on their own emotions, thoughts, aspirations, experiences, work and relationships, it's very unlikely they'll be focusing on your tummy. And if they do ever make a nasty comment, they're probably not someone you should waste your time worrying about anyway. But in the ten years I've had IBS, I've never had a nasty comment about my tummy noises. In fact, when I now talk to people

I used to sit next to in school, who I worried could hear my tummy, I've found out they were none the wiser.

Don't let it be a distraction

If you think these noises are going to cause you a distraction from important exams or meetings, take action to make yourself feel as comfortable as possible. For example, I paid for a doctor's note to explain the situation to my teachers. I asked for a special arrangement to be made so that I could sit all of my exams in a separate room to my peers. That way, I wouldn't have to worry about my stomach noises affecting anyone else and I could concentrate purely on the work in hand. I could also leave if I needed to go to the loo at any given moment, without anyone saying anything because there was no-one to comment. I wouldn't recommend this in EVERY situation because I do think it's good to not shy away from what you're afraid of but if you really think it's going to be of detriment to your grades, it may be an option worth considering.

Hydrate yourself

Sip water, slowly. Sometimes this in itself can 'drown' the angry alien on the rollercoaster as it relaxes the gut and stops it spasming.

Learn what the alien likes to eat and doesn't like

We will talk about food in greater depth in different chapters, but I will touch upon this briefly in the context of stomach noises. It is a good idea to reduce foods that cause gas. I know that I'm more prone to tummy noises if I eat certain foods. When I cut out dairy, this eliminated about 80% of the sounds. However, I also know that more acidic foods cause my tummy to growl. I love clementines and oranges, but they make my stomach sing. So if I'm going into a quiet situation afterwards, I'll avoid them or explain that my stomach is auditioning for *Britain's Got Talent*.

Don't encourage the alien

We'll talk more about anxiety causing flare-ups, but if you find that you are often worried about your stomach making a noise which, in turn, means it does make a noise – then you could be stuck in a negative cycle that can feel very difficult and overwhelming to escape from.

In this book, I hope to provide a range of tried and tested options for you to try that will help minimise particular symptoms and hopefully help alleviate the impact they are having on your life. To start with, however, we'll go into how IBS can affect each aspect of your daily life, and then we'll work our way into the realms of some potential solutions.

Many people underestimate the emotional toll that IBS can have on an individual and how isolating a condition it can be.

I naively thought that when I received my initial IBS diagnosis, my months of turmoil and tears would finally come to a sweet 'normal poo' end.

But alas, it was only just the beginning of a very confusing, anxious journey which has ultimately led me here.

CHAPTER 2

Anxiety

I remember the doctor's words as he eliminated the possibility of it being Crohn's, UC or IBD.

"Scarlett, it's JUST IBS."

He handed me a pamphlet with a toilet on the front of it, which briefly summarised the somewhat 'trivial' sounding symptoms of IBS.

I was so confused; how could something that affected me so drastically every day be ONLY IBS?

Surely, they must have made a mistake.

Where on earth did I go from here?

I think the lack of a solution sent me into a downward spiral for the first couple of months. I felt so hopeless that I'd have to live with this awful condition for the rest of my life without any apparent cure on the horizon.

Anxiety is a very real symptom of IBS and a very real trigger too.

I found myself worrying about having an IBS flare-up, which would, in turn, CAUSE an IBS flare-up because our gut and our brains are so closely intertwined.

Our gut is apparently our second brain and so it reacts physically to the hormones produced by our emotions. It's a total catch-22 situation.

Similarly, anxiety and periods of stress that are unrelated to our tummies can also cause the symptoms. In fact, I truly believe it was a period of particularly stressful exam pressure at school that actually caused my IBS to start in the first place.

I'll never forget my first episode of an IBS attack.

It was the last lesson of the day and I was the envy of my classmates as I had been sat next to the boy who every girl in my year happened to have a huge crush on. I was feeling rather smug that I'd bagged the best seat in the house.

I was also super excited about the lesson itself, which was Media Studies, a new subject at our school that I was SURE

I was going to love. This was partly due to *Friends* having been featured on the pamphlet, and as a result I had convinced myself we'd be watching back-to-back episodes for the duration. Spoiler: it didn't happen.

But regardless, I guess you could say there was a certain excited energy inside me that afternoon, giddy that I'd bagged a seat next to the guy everyone was crushing on and also that it wasn't another boring Maths lesson.

I was going through a stressful time, with an exam period looming and teachers piling on the pressure, but I was excited about this lesson in particular.

Perhaps it was a mix of the excitement - which your body can sometimes mistake for anxiety - have you ever been excited about a holiday, but felt sick with nerves instead - they both incite the production of adrenaline so sometimes your body can get a little confused. Unfortunately, that day marked my first experience of an IBS attack. And it was pretty hideous.

About five minutes after sitting down and the class starting, a slightly heavy feeling started in my lower stomach. The same feeling you get when you get an urge to go to the loo. But only this was immediate and felt VERY URGENT.

Our school had a rule that you couldn't go to the toilet once the class had started, so I knew that I wasn't going to be able to relieve the urge immediately. This, in itself, panicked me, as I'd never had SUCH an overwhelming urge to go to the loo before.

In the next three minutes, my stomach started making crazy noises that I'd never experienced before.

It sounded like my stomach was actually FARTING, loudly and ferociously. The sensation rollercoastered up and down, and the noises followed suit. I had a sharp pain in the right side of my stomach that felt like I needed to expel wind, only it never actually reached the 'exit' and, instead, quickly rollercoastered back inside me and made an almighty noise.

I was absolutely MORTIFIED. How on earth could my body let me down in such a hideous way?

I had absolutely NO control over what was happening. And worst of all, it was extremely painful.

I felt a surge of hot sweaty panic through my body and all of a sudden, the room I was in – *a classroom where I'd spent many hundreds of hours throughout my life previously* – felt VERY scary, intimidating and overwhelming.

I did a good job of hiding and muffling the situation that ensued, and if I'm honest, I have absolutely NO idea how on earth I got through the next hour. I just remember bursting out the door and running to my mum's car before breaking down in tears.

Together, we concluded that I must have had food poisoning or consumed too many fruit smoothies that morning, and I took the following day off school.

But it happened again. And again. And soon I realised that even going to the loo (and reacting to that initial urge) wouldn't necessarily stop it from happening.

I began to develop an anxiety disorder and phobia of being in quiet, confined spaces. The thought of stepping into a lecture theatre, or a classroom, or a meeting where I couldn't easily excuse myself without causing attention, would fill me with a sense of impending dread.

I think if you'd asked me whether I'd rather have sat in a tank full of snakes and spiders, or set foot in a classroom again, I'd have picked the bloody spiders.

And I HATE spiders.

Some part of this deep-rooted anxiety remains still inside me even now. I hate it if I'm in a quiet room with people who don't know about my IBS and someone closes the door. It's like a switch inside me is flicked.

Hot, sweaty panic rises inside of me. My breathing and heart rate increases and the room starts spinning. I start to feel hideously sick in the pit of my stomach, which suddenly starts gurgling away.

I guess part of it is that I'm worried that other people can hear what's going on inside my stomach and somehow 'reveal' me to the world. And part of me is so frustrated that my body is letting me down in such a way.

But I know there is a way out of this cycle and the anxiety-inducing moments that IBS might be causing.

I've since tried hypnotherapy, counselling, anti-depressants, beta-blockers and CBT to stop this anxious cycle from happening. And I've had varying levels of success with each one.

I'm not going to lie to you and say that I'm 'cured' or that it disappeared miraculously one day because there have been three occasions over the past year when I've had this hideous panic attack cycle. Once when I was at a dinner at a friend's house, once during a press conference where the A-List actress Jennifer Lawrence was standing in front of me, and another time when I was attending a product launch and there was a quiet PowerPoint presentation beforehand. But I now have the tools to stop these panic attacks from manifesting and halt them in their tracks before they can cause any issues.

I credit CBT to most of this, as 'Cognitive Behavioural Therapy' is all about retraining and realigning your thought processes to not immediately jump to a conclusion, i.e. not immediately worrying about my IBS flaring up JUST because I'm in a quiet situation. Just because it's happened in the past, doesn't mean it will happen again.

It is based on the premise that our view of the world is shaped by our previous experiences. This is a very normal habit, which has shaped us up until this point. As a child, we learn right from wrong. This helps us to grow up and become independent. It harks back to us at our most primitive, as mechanically we are made to use our 'fight or flight' response. In the animal world, they use their previous experiences and instincts to either fight (tackle the situation – attack) or flight (run away and hide). This is a basic instinct that helps them to survive. But in the human world, we perceive many situations in the same way.

For example, being afraid of cats can often be linked to an experience you've had in the past. You may have been attacked by a cat as a child. You experienced pain as a result of a scratch and have therefore associated cats with pain. And therefore, a fear of cats ensued as a result. Obviously, not everyone will process the situation in the same way. Many will have endured a cat scratch and known it's not a reason to be afraid of ALL cats, full stop. But we all process situations differently. They shape our instincts, our thoughts and how we process situations.

CBT is about retraining and reshaping immediate thought patterns that respond to certain stimuli.

One thing that helps massively is to have a list of questions on standby to 'ask yourself internally' when those immediate reactions start, i.e. if you see a cat

CBT also recommends 'exposure therapy' as part of your recovery process. So rather than avoiding doing something for long periods of time, and therefore making the fear worse, they recommend you should gently expose yourself to the fear - and gradually increase this over time, i.e. if you were afraid of cats, perhaps a recommendation would be to sit near a cat for two minutes. And then gradually build this up.

There are many great books out there that I'd recommend you read if you are genuinely interested in trying out CBT for yourself. These explain the premise of CBT in far greater depth (and more eloquently) than I have attempted to. CBT is something you'll have to put some real time and effort into for a period of time and the results aren't always instantaneous, but it's had some fantastic results, and I am testament to how much it has helped me over time.

If you're based in the UK, there is a self-referral you can do on the internet to enquire about free help and CBT sessions. You can also pay for private sessions, of course, which usually have more flexibility and freedom. Sessions can generally cost anywhere between £25 and £80, depending on who you go to. Sometimes, you may have to 'shop around' to find someone you are comfortable with because CBT is only really effective when you talk to someone you can let your guard down with. Not everyone is going to feel right with the same person, so don't feel bad if the first therapist you see isn't the right one for you. Depending on where you live, you may need to get a referral from your GP to be eligible for CBT on the NHS, or you may be able to self-refer online. The local wellbeing service I used was called 'Steps2Wellbeing'; however, if you Google 'wellbeing services in INSERT WHERE YOU LIVE HERE', you'll usually be able to find out more information.

If you don't feel comfortable seeing a therapist and you'd prefer to try CBT at home, there are many online resources, courses and books you can try. From personal experience, I found a few sessions of talking to a physical person very helpful, just to get me started with CBT; however, many therapists offer Skype consultations or telephone assessments if you're more comfortable with that.

At the end of the book, I've listed a few resources and books that I found immensely helpful.

Often anxiety isn't something that just goes away on its own, and nor will it ever disappear forever. Anxiety is a normal, natural thing and a little bit of anxiety is actually GOOD for us, as it means we care. It means we are conscientious individuals. It means we are creative and hard-working. But when it overwhelms us and causes something like IBS to flare-up, it's got out of hand and we need to do something about it.

Whether you're a naturally anxious person or whether it's developed as a result of IBS, it will need to be worked on by you on a regular basis. Just as we have to exercise our bodies and keep it healthy and fit, our minds also need work and to be treated kindly.

Mindfulness can be really helpful at calming yourself down when you are in the face of a 'fight or flight' situation because it helps to bring your mind to the 'present' moment rather than letting your head fill up with emotions, thoughts, pre-conceived ideas and previous experiences; pre-empting what's going to happen. If you do start to feel yourself panicking, here are some handy tips:

Focus

Take a sip of water and gently swallow it, focusing on the sensation of the water trickling down your throat. Before taking the next sip, take a deep breath, inhaling slowly inwards and then deeply outwards.

Ground yourself

Take your shoes off and let your feet touch the ground. This may sound strange but it's really helped me during moments of sheer panic. 'Grounding yourself' in this very literal way can help you to regain control of your thoughts and focus on the present moment. This is particularly helpful if you're outdoors, though I wouldn't recommend this particular tip if it's winter. And it's muddy outside.

A trip to the mind zoo

Count to twenty, in elephant form. Or whatever your favourite animal is. One ELEPHANT. Two ELEPHANT. As you count, make sure that you take deep breaths in between each elephant, or llama or kangaroo (anything BUT tarantula, let's face it). The insertion of an animal helps to take your mind into a more positive realm and also elongates the counting, so you are focusing solely on each count and each breath.

Ride the rollercoaster

Instead of panicking when you feel the emotions start to overwhelm you, tell yourself that you're excited to 'ride the coaster'. I sometimes find it's a help to plaster a huge smile on my face, which confuses my brain and my body, and melts away the 'panic instinct'. It sounds silly, but can sometimes really work wonders!

Channel your energy elsewhere

If, like me, you have always been quite an anxious and sensitive individual, then we might be duped into thinking this side of us is a 'flaw'. But, as I've said above, being this way is actually a positive thing. We are anxious because we often overthink. And we often overthink because we care. We are conscientious, caring and kind people who put external pressures onto ourselves to achieve, to please others and to succeed. We may have big dreams, hopes for the future and we give a lot of ourselves to our friends. However, a lot of our energy is spent on worrying, which isn't productive and is often a total waste of our time and adrenaline. So one of my top tips is to try and channel that energy into something else. Distract your 100mph mind and find something you LOVE doing. For me, this was writing – and my blog. Now, if I'm ever feeling worried or very anxious, I'll open up a notebook and write away. It really helps me to clear my mind, get my thoughts down on paper and stop them from manifesting into things that cause IBS symptoms. Perhaps yours could be a sport or taking up a new activity, like crochet, drawing, painting or gardening.

Fact or opinion

If my mind REALLY gets carried away with itself, I often have to press a metaphorical 'pause' button and ask myself 'is this a fact or an opinion'. For example, if I worry what people will think about me when I have to leave the room to dash to the toilet, I might be thinking 'they are going to laugh, stare, talk behind my back and think less of me'. But is there proof behind this statement? Chances are there probably isn't. It's an opinion. Your own biased opinion. Your own judgement and it's really not worth wasting your energy on. I'm not saying your judgement is irrelevant, but we do have to be strong with ourselves sometimes and question whether our own minds are running away with themselves. Usually, we do this because we are creatively minded and imaginative. So again, try channelling that creativity elsewhere.

Face the fear

This is definitely a technique that I am still working on and is the most difficult but effective way to combat the fear and anxiety surrounding IBS. For example, my fear of being in a room that I can't easily escape from. I could choose to avoid situations like these forever more, or I could opt to never sit in a quiet room again or attend a meeting without background noise. But by pandering to this fear, I am essentially growing it. By avoiding these situations, I am allowing that irrational fear to grow inside me like poison ivy and get stronger and stronger. So I make sure that I DO face these situations from time to time, in a controlled environment. And what has happened? Well, at first I panicked, hated it and let the fear overwhelm me. But after breathing through those initial five minutes, the rest seemed like a breeze. It's important that we don't succumb to our fears and let them manifest themselves and control our lives. I never wanted to let my IBS stop me from achieving my dreams. At many points, it almost did. But small steps can be taken to slowly conquer that fear, and this is something you can work through individually with a therapist or by using CBT techniques.

Find a calming motion

This is a technique that I learned during a hypnotherapy session several years ago and it's really helped me during the moments that lead up to me having a panic attack. In fact, I've successfully used it (even recently) to halt a panic attack in its tracks and restore a calm mind. It involves finding a repetitive small movement that you can do to slow down your mind and your breathing. For me, I take my forefinger and my index finger on my right hand and rub them in circular motions on the open flattened palm of my left hand. It not only feels quite relaxing, but I find this simple motion can really help me to 'ground' myself, slow down my mind and my breathing and stop the panic from gaining momentum. I was recently in a workshop with my boyfriend in Amsterdam when suddenly, the door to the room closed and the room was totally silent. As you'll know from the rest of the book, this was my nightmare. I felt the panic start to rise, got all hot and sweaty and my breathing became rapid and shallow. But I started the circular motions on the palm of my hand, counted my elephants and within a minute, I felt fine. Often I can let panic run away with me; it's about stopping it in its tracks and slowing down.

Breath through your belly

There's something you do over 25,000 times a day without even thinking about it – breathing. But actually, harnessing our awareness to our breath can be a hugely helpful way of de-stressing, reducing panic attacks and generally boosting your positive wellbeing. As a quick exercise, put one hand on your chest now and the other on your belly (sorry, I haven't quite factored in which hand is going to hold this book – maybe you could balance it between your toes) and inhale deeply, before exhaling. Notice which hand moves more – is it the hand on your chest or the one on your belly? Chances are it's the one on your chest because, typically, most adults tend to breathe through their chest, which is a habit learned from prolonged periods of stress. Most young children, on the other hand (who are typically far more carefree and stress-free, as they haven't learned bad habits) breathe naturally through their belly. Try to breathe again, and this time, do it through your belly. Do this quietly on your own 10-15 times and notice how relaxed you feel afterwards. This really worked for me and I practice 'belly' breathing whenever I'm feeling particularly anxious.

SAMANTHA'S STORY

Samantha Hearne is a wonderful anxiety and business coach who has hosted workshops at some of the previous networking events that I have put together. She radiates such positive energy and is a pleasure to be around. In fact, I'd go as far as to say that I am instantly reassured in her presence (both online and IRL). She has also suffered from IBS and was kind enough to share her journey with me for this book. If you'd like to find out more about Samantha or chat to her about coaching, visit her website 'A Happy Mind'.

Do you have your own personal affinity with IBS? Was it something you suffered from yourself personally? And can you explain the journey you went through with it?

Yes, I did struggle with IBS for the majority of my twenties. Anxiety was huge for me and this was the biggest contributing factor for my IBS.

I used to struggle to go to the toilet when anyone else was around, in the house or nearby. I couldn't be rushed and could never just 'go' when I needed to. I had to have complete peace – in my mind, my surroundings and with time. Anxiety made me feel tense and stressed a lot of the time, as well as emotional, and this hugely impacted my IBS. It was very emotionally led and this was something that took me a long time to realise.

I would notice patterns with the IBS too. Travelling was a no-go! I would go at least 24 hours before being able to go to the toilet and if I had to get up early, travel anywhere or go out before I was ready, I just had to hold it in and this caused me so much pain. I would even have to wake up earlier than I needed so that I had time to just sit on the toilet without panicking or rushing.

Once I had mastered my anxiety and started to change my mindset, the IBS started to subside and I was able to move forward past this stage of worry and stress.

This, of course, takes time. My biggest advice would be to look deeper than the surface level 'problems' and see if you can unpick the trends, the worries and the external factors that impact the IBS.

How can someone who feels beaten by their IBS symptoms take steps to get into a happier and more positive frame of mind?

You can 100% work around it and need to focus on all the things that you CAN do.

Self-care is huge and taking time for yourself daily – or weekly at a minimum – to reset your mind, your body and find a balance when you need it most. These slices of time will just allow you to genuinely find calm in amongst the manic, hectic days you may experience.

Diet and wellbeing are key too. For me, alcohol was a big issue, so I stopped drinking so much and became the driver. I could still socialise and have fun, but I also had the freedom to leave if I needed to and be in control of the situation.

If you know certain foods/drinks/substances affect the IBS for you, then find adaptations that you can make to better your health.

Allow yourself time to regroup. When the IBS does flair-up or seems worse, allow yourself the time to get back on track. Don't push yourself too hard. The more effort you put into 'pretending to be OK,' the longer lasting the pain will be it can cause you.

Find support and wisdom from those around you – podcasts, books, blogs. You are not an alien and should never feel isolated by the IBS. So surround yourself with people that can empathise and support you, in the ways you would support them.

What coping techniques would you recommend to someone who is suffering from IBS?

Deep breathing and relaxation are HUGE for me – even now!

If I am due on, this affects my bowels and I also still struggle with travel and being able to go to the toilet. So deep breathing and relaxation time are MASSIVE for me!

One simple tip is to balance your in and out breath, so that they match. If you breathe in for a count of 4, do the same for your out breath and just focus on this. Focus on your breathing and find a natural balance for yourself.

Hot baths are my best friend too! So if you are finding it hard to de-stress and physically relax your body, find something that can help you to do this. Baths were the answer for me.

I find IBS and anxiety to be a catch-22 situation, as worrying about having a flare-up can often cause it. In your experience, how does IBS affect and cause anxiety?

The more you think about it, the more likely it is to happen.

If you are sending your energy and focus to something that 'could' happen, the likelihood is it will.

You are just as likely not to have a flare-up today, as you are to have one.

As an anxiety coach, I deal with this a lot, and I now use these two questions to help combat this:

O   HAS IT HAPPENED YET? **(NO!)**

O   COULD I FOCUS ON SOMETHING POSITIVE INSTEAD **(YES)**

The brackets are the answers that usually come up and this is what I reinforce into my thinking as often as I need to. Have a go at this yourself!

Although I've suffered from IBS for over 10 years now, I feel it blew up into a full-blown anxiety disorder at university when I was hundreds of miles away from home, without my immediate support systems in place and a lot of added pressure on my plate. For me, the main anxiety is being in enclosed spaces, so I start to panic and sweat (and then my stomach starts making angry alien noises) whenever someone closes the door of a meeting room and I can't easily excuse myself if I need to dash to the toilet. It seems to have developed into an almost irrational fear, as I hate being in quiet enclosed spaces. What techniques would you recommend to be the most effective for me? And is this something you find in a lot of IBS patients?

Having irrational fears and worries is a common struggle with anxiety and fear. Again, I would start with breathing techniques. This is your most powerful resource and you have it with you everywhere you go, so take full advantage of that!

On top of that, I think the key thing is to externalise these fears. The more you hold them within you, the more powerful and poisonous they become. So share them with someone you love and trust and allow them to help you pacify and rationalise, until you are strong enough to do this for yourself. Don't keep these worries within, or they will continue to take hold of you – share them, reduce them and stop taking ownership of them.

IBS can be quite socially isolating, as the symptoms can be unrelenting and cause you to stay at home. Do you have any advice for those suffering from the social isolation aspect?

Simple. Allow yourself the time to rest and recover.

It can be hard to miss out and not be able to be as social as you want, but the more you focus on these down points and the things that you 'can't do', the longer the stress and tension build up within. Be honest with yourself and if you need time to rest, take it!

The right people will always give you the right support and love.

I can't pinpoint one particular trigger of my IBS. I just know I've always been very sensitive and my stomach seems to be my 'health flaw' that is affected whenever things get too much. Is there any way that I can retrain myself not to let all my anxieties go straight to my 'symptoms'?

O   TRY TO REFRAME THE THOUGHT

O   THE ANXIETY WON'T LEAD TO THE PHYSICAL PAIN

O   THE ANXIETY AND THOUGHTS ARE NOT PHYSICAL

O   THE THOUGHTS AND FEARS DO NOT NEED TO BECOME PHYSICAL

O   MY THOUGHTS ARE NOT MY PHYSICAL BODY

These statements can be really helpful in reframing these anxieties.

I must say, all of this takes time and consistency, but it 100% worked for me and has changed my life, so I love sharing these steps with all of you.

Remember, you are not alone. You are not an alien and things CAN and WILL improve for you.

LOOK DEEPER THAN THE SURFACE LEVEL

'PROBLEMS' AND SEE IF YOU CAN UNPICK

THE TRENDS, THE WORRIES AND THE

EXTERNAL FACTORS THAT IMPACT THE IBS.

"Eat to make your body happy."

What goes in, must come out, as they rather unsympathetically say. And as IBS sufferers, don't we know it!

CHAPTER 3

Food

When I was 14 and newly diagnosed, my doctor advised me to try a dairy-free diet for a month to see if my symptoms would improve somewhat.

He advised me to keep a food diary to try and identify any triggers before then sending me on my merry way, into the scary world of potential food intolerances.

In 2019, it's fairly easy to lead this kind of temporary elimination diet, with an abundance of options available to us in our local supermarkets in the 'Free From' aisle; however, back in 2006, it was a different story.

Dairy seemed to feature in EVERYTHING and there wasn't much in the way of plant-based alternatives.

I remember once sobbing into a bag of prawn cocktail crisps slumped against the fridge because I realised I couldn't have them anymore.

They were jam-packed with milk powder, even if they looked relatively dairy-free friendly.

This not only illustrated my tendency to be slightly overdramatic, but also made me realise I was going to have to give up my normal routine to try and fix this new problem. How unfair, why me?

Looking back, I wasn't ready to weigh up what was more important – 'Scarlett potentially feeling better' or 'Scarlett having her crisps and eating them' – but it was my first real taste (excuse the pun) of how food could affect my symptoms.

Admittedly, I didn't stick to it in the way I should have and therefore didn't see much of a difference, so at my next appointment, my doctor suggested that I try a gluten-free diet instead.

This was much easier, but also fairly intimidating, especially as a 14-year-old who was trying to maintain a social life and keep up with friends.

I was known as the 'gluten-free' girl for a couple of months, carrying around my pot of gluten-free tomato pasta in an 'uncool' Tupperware container, while my friends popped to the canteen for pizza and cake.

They didn't have to think about preparing something special beforehand. Nor did they have to be the awkward one at social gatherings requesting gluten-free bread.

I begrudged my dysfunctional stomach yet again.

Though there was a slight improvement, I wasn't sobbing into bagels.

As hideous as my IBS was, clearly the pain and the discomfort was not enough for me at that point to truly stick to an elimination diet and figure out my triggers once and for all. And so, the symptoms ensued.

It wasn't until I was 21 and hundreds of miles away from home at university that I finally had enough of an incentive to find out exactly what food was doing to my body and how it was affecting my IBS symptoms once and for all.

I was at the point where I was being woken up in the middle of the night, every night, in agonising pain with my stomach.

I couldn't leave the house without having twelve toilet trips beforehand - and even then, I'd fear for more. At my absolute worst, I was practically bedbound (or bathroom-bound) and far too poorly to attend lectures because I couldn't keep anything in my stomach and was so exhausted from all the turmoil.

I would ring the non-emergency number almost once a week, retailing my symptoms to the phone operator, slightly hoping she'd send an ambulance for me because I was convinced that the excruciating pain was the result of something far more sinister.

Surely this couldn't be 'just IBS'.

My then-boyfriend would watch in turmoil as I sobbed all night long from the stabbing pains in my stomach, which felt like a sharp knife was being twisted through my intestines repeatedly.

I know I'm a tad overdramatic, but trust me, there was no other way to describe this agonising pain.

It was absolutely hideous and I wouldn't wish this on my worst enemy (not that I have a worst enemy, but you know the phrase); however, getting to this point was probably the best thing that ever happened to me because it incentivised me to finally tackle my issues head-on and get to the bottom of what was going on. Excuse the pun.

I couldn't live the rest of my life like this – surely there was another way.

I couldn't put my life on hold because my stomach couldn't figure out what it was doing.

So I used my time while bedbound to research all things IBS related.

I discovered that food was a huge factor affecting digestive symptoms and that common triggers were dairy and gluten, as the doctor had advised me almost ten years prior.

I took a food intolerance test (with York Test) which flagged dairy and eggs as big triggers for me and overnight, I cut them out of my diet completely.

I know many people are cynical of food intolerance testing however speaking from personal experience, it gave me a starting point for what to cut out first, as the online FODMAP list (we'll talk about this later) was never-ending and rather daunting.

I paid close attention to food labels because dairy seemed to be a sneaky ingredient for many unrelated products.

Summer Fruits Rose wine, salt & vinegar crisps, risottos, shop-bought guacamole and soups were just some of the crazy discoveries I made along the way that contained whey powder, casein (a milk protein) or cream.

Even today, when chatting to new people about my dairy-free diet, there is a standard response of: "Oh yes, well I don't eat much dairy either."

But most of the world eat far more than they think because it's hidden in so many different items.

Let's look at the average day-to-day diet of a person in the UK.

○ BREAKFAST: CEREAL & MILK.

Usually, the cereal will contain some form of dairy (i.e. Special K) and then, of course, you have the milk too.

○ LUNCH: SANDWICH WITH FILLING.

Usually, sandwiches contain butter, some sort of cheese product and also a sauce. Mayo contains egg, salad cream contains – you guessed it – cream.

○ DINNER: LASAGNE/SAUSAGE & MASH/PASTA/ RISOTTO.

A lot of pre-made pasta sauces contain dairy, mashed potato contains butter, risotto contains cream, butter and often parmesan.

And that's just a small selection of common meals.

My point is that because triggers are snuck into so many of our favourite dishes, there are often grey areas as to what might be setting off your symptoms.

Not everyone with IBS will have the same triggers, which is why it's important to really keep track of your symptoms and what foods you're consuming on a day-to-day basis.

Sometimes you can pinpoint specific things. For example, if you usually eat very plain food on an everyday basis and then go out with friends and have a pizza, your symptoms may get worse the next day or immediately after eating.

However, it usually takes a period of 3-6 months of extensively monitoring what foods agree with you or don't to draw definitive conclusions about what might be helping or making your symptoms worse.

At the end of the book, I have provided a simple food diary set-up that I used in these very telling first few months to track what I was eating and what kind of a reaction it was having on my body.

As well as improving my IBS symptoms drastically, there was the added benefit of becoming far more in tune with my body and working in harmony with it by listening to it, in order to keep it happy and working properly.

Not everyone will have the same intolerances forever, so in many cases, it's worth keeping a food diary indefinitely; however, I'd give all new patterns of eating at least 1-3 months before I'd expect to see a noticeable difference in your symptoms.

For me, a turning point was week 3, when I noticed that my toilet trips had normalised from 12 a day, to 1 or 2.

While I still had a few IBS type bouts, it was a million times better than when I was at my lowest, and so for this reason, I do stick to a strict dairy-free, egg-free diet on a permanent basis.

Some people are happy to have 'cheat' days where they indulge in their favourite creamy desserts and 'suffer the consequences' afterwards, but for me, those consequences simply aren't worth a temporary sweet tooth satiation.

There are so many wonderful and more nutritious plant-based alternatives, I'm happy to go without.

Cutting out dairy and eggs was a daunting process for me initially, because before doing so, you would not have been surprised if I'd changed my middle name to 'Parmesan' – I literally ate cheese for breakfast, lunch and dinner.

However, it was an easy decision to make when I realised how much of a better quality life I would have without it in my tummy.

There were also some surprising additional perks of cutting out dairy. These came in the form of an unexpected three stone drop in weight over the period of a year and my skin (which had been plagued by rosacea for so many years) also cleared up.

My BMI was slightly high before cutting out dairy (which may or may not have been because I inhaled family-sized bars of Galaxy Caramel every night, straight after a large bowl of cheesy pasta), and I went from 11 stone 6 to 8 stone 6 within 12 months.

These days, I do try to use food as my medicine (more on medicine later) because I know how much of an effect (positive or negative) it can have on our bodies.

Another common IBS food trigger detection process is a diet called the 'Low FODMAP Plan', which asks you to completely eliminate foods that are high in fermentable short-chain sugars called FODMAPs.

A lot of research has been conducted into this diet and the results have been very positive, so it's a very popular starting point that many doctors recommend.

Once again, it can be extremely daunting initially as the list of foods you 'cannot eat' is as long as the list that you can.

When I initially starting trying this diet and almost burst into tears in the supermarket because I was so overwhelmed by how many things had garlic or onion in them.

However with some careful planning and lots of home-cooking, it can be done. It is a great way to very specifically pinpoint what could be setting off your symptoms; as in some cases, different foods can cause very different symptoms.

After an elimination period, one-by-one you slowly start to reintroduce different foods back into your diet, all while closely monitoring your symptoms.

For me, I know that chickpeas cause a lot of puffiness and gas, whereas dairy gives me diarrhoea, brings me out in a rash and leaves me feeling very exhausted within a couple of hours of eating it.

Onions and garlic can leave me feeling a tad bloated, but it is not usually bad enough to strictly cut them out entirely.

Onions seem to fare worse for me than garlic, the latter of which I LOVE in chicken dishes, so I'm quite grateful it doesn't cause too much of a reaction.

It totally depends on the individual and what kind of a reaction each food induces.

The solution for your particular symptoms lies in doing as much research as possible and then implementing a trial and error type of programme. There categorically IS going to be something that works for you. A management plan is definitely out there, it's just waiting for you to find it. And it might not be the first thing you try, or the second or the third. In my case, it took almost eight years of trial and error.

It's also very important to employ the help of an expert whenever you're changing your eating patterns because it can be unhealthy to cut out entire food groups unnecessarily (as you're not getting the nutrients you need) and potentially dangerous (because restrictive eating can spiral into eating disorders).

I recently discovered a very interesting podcast by the Doctor's Kitchen and Dr Alan Desmond (I would highly recommend you have a listen), which was all about eating in the right way to promote gut health.

I was astounded by some of the facts and figures they presented, including that 55% of the calories that we consume in the UK come from processed foods which don't have any nutrients or fibre in them.

And subsequently, many of us aren't hitting the required 30g of fibre on a day-to-day basis. In fact, lots of us aren't reaching anywhere near that.

Fibre is vital for IBS sufferers and although the quantity you should have depends on a number of different factors (how much you eat during the day, your age, your weight etc), those who suffer from both constipation and diarrhoea need to make sure they're getting the RIGHT kind of fibre in their diet.

It took me a while to get my head around the two types of fibre – soluble and insoluble. Insoluble – like its name suggests – is not broken down in the gut, but it does add bulk to your waste (i.e. poo) which helps to keep you regular and prevents constipation. You're likely to find insoluble fibre in roughage items, such as the skin of vegetables, wholegrains, nuts and fruit.

Meanwhile, soluble fibre is sticky and soft and absorbs water to form a gel-like texture, which assists in softening your poo. The softer the poo, the more easily it can slide through the digestive tract and bind waste material, clearing out your system. It also helps to absorb nutrients into the bloodstream, so it's amazing for your health and, apparently, it boosts the population of good bacteria in your gut too. Win-win! You'll find this kind of fibre in beans, avocado, peas and oats, and it's said to keep you fuller for longer and more satisfied after meal-times, so you're not reaching for anything sugary to satiate a craving!

Some foods, such as lentils, contain both soluble and insoluble fibre, so it's important to get a real mix in order to keep things moving and provide much-needed harmony to your digestive system. I found that often my diarrhoea could be linked to when I had been eating greasy food that was lacking in nutrition. I then needed the fibre to bulk things up and slow down the movement of waste through my digestive system.

At the very end of the book, I have provided a list of additional resources that I would personally recommend you have a look into. They are a means of providing the best possible foundations for you to ensure the food that you're putting into your body will be harmonious with your digestive system and create the best possible basis for your IBS management.

TIPS

Eating out

Eating out when you're going through an elimination diet can be a tricky and daunting expedition, but it's by no means impossible, it just takes a bit of extra planning.

If you know the name of the restaurant you'll be visiting, either log onto their website or ring ahead to see what's on offer.

Most places offer special menus to cater for a variety of different dietary requirements, and don't forget, they want you to have a good time and enjoy your food as a guest of theirs, so don't feel like you're being a nuisance or being awkward. Anything but!

If you're dining in a foreign country, make sure that you get free business cards (Vistaprint offer free business card printing) stating your intolerances or dietary requirements in the local language. This then eliminates you having to awkwardly explain (or in my previous cases, mime with lots of gesticulation) at the dinner table, what you can and can't eat. You simply hand over the card!

If in doubt, stick to plain food. Most places will grill you a chicken breast and cook you some plain white rice if you request it.

Take it back to basics

Occasionally, I will go through a week or so where ANY food I eat sets off my symptoms. I could be eating plain oats, rice and chicken and I'll still have a painful bloated gassy stomach that feels like someone has stuffed a basketball inside my intestines and is still trying to pump it up. Not comfortable, whatsoever.

I think that when it comes to IBS, food isn't always the main trigger, which means that even though certain aspects of your diet might set you off, there may be other, overriding triggers that are non-food related. Perhaps you're going through a particularly stressful period at work (or you've just come through the other side of it; sometimes, symptoms can be delayed and the stress takes its toll later on down the line), or maybe you're deficient in certain minerals and vitamins.

It can be quite defeating when you've restricted your food and it STILL isn't enough for your stubborn IBS symptoms, however, try not to let it get you down and listen to your body as much as you can. Perhaps it needs to have some TLC in other areas. More on this later.

When you're going through periods like this, I find it helpful to try and stick to very plain, low-fibre foods. White bread toast, white rice, plain chicken and plain crackers. You WILL come through the other side, I promise! If you're struggling during a period like this, make sure you check out my 'recipes' section at the end for some of my fail-safe IBS-friendly meal plans!

Figure out your transit time

Everyone has a different transit time (i.e. the time it takes for the food you put in to actually come out) and it's worth sometimes testing to see what yours is like. This way, you'll know how quickly it's going to take for food to potentially produce a symptom or present an issue.

For me, my transit time is 24 hours. However, others may need to go to the loo just an hour after eating. A way of figuring this out is to eat a portion of sweetcorn in your next meal and then time how long it takes for it to reappear in your toilet bowl. Super gross, perhaps, but interesting, as it's really helpful information that will make you a little bit more in tune with your own body.

Being in sync with yourself is an amazing blessing that I – weirdly – have IBS to thank for because it motivated me to do so. I now know so much about my body and can predict how it will react to almost anything. It also allows me to regain some of the control that IBS so graciously takes away from us.

Get into a routine

One thing that helped me immensely in the early days of IBS was to get myself into a routine that my body and bowel habits could get used to. I began having porridge and peppermint tea as soon as I woke up in the morning (7am), as I found that the hot food would set my bowels into gear and so I'd be able to have a poo before I left the house. That way, I felt reassured that I'd had one bowel movement in the comfort of my own home and could feel a little more 'normal' in myself, again regaining some of that control that I felt had been ripped away from me.

I had a cold but filling and nutritious lunch around 1pm and then dinner at 5pm, so as to give it enough time to properly digest before heading to bed. If I felt the need to snack, I'd have an oat bar around 11am and 3pm. I also tended to eat smaller portions as to not overload my stomach with food and cause pain.

Getting into a routine was extremely beneficial for controlling my symptoms and it is still something I do today. Even when I travel for work, I tend to stick to the exact same routine whenever possible, but I do it in the new time zone. Your body adjusts quicker than you think!

Try Intermittent Fasting

If you're really struggling and having a tough time with your symptoms, then I would recommend looking into intermittent fasting. This technique was actually introduced to me by my nutritionist and I was astounded at just how much it helped me.

Fasting has received a bit of a bad rep in the diet world (largely because there's so much misinformation about it) but it can be a really effective way to give your digestion an extended break, allowing it to heal and recover, which can really help to alleviate symptoms.

Try to keep your eating to an 8-hour window. So if you have your first meal at 9am, you have your last morsel of food no later than 5pm. Then you have a 16-hour fasting window which gives your digestion a rest. It sounds daunting but as long as you're eating plenty of nutritious, healthy, wholesome food in your eight-hour window, you shouldn't be hungry during your fasting window.

Drink plenty of water

Keeping your body hydrated has SO many benefits and for IBS sufferers, there are even more perks to drinking enough water.

For one, it keeps things moving in your body and it flushes out your system. It also helps to treat and prevent constipation because it stops your waste product from drying out and, therefore, becoming sluggish in the bowel.

I also found sipping water gently and regularly throughout the day minimised those angry, windy growls that used to crop up during the most AWKWARD of timings. Quiet meeting + a stomach that sounds like a whistling farty alien on a rollercoaster = one embarrassed Scarlett. Water keeps the alien at bay. I always keep a bottle with me at all times. I also find sipping on water can be immensely helpful when encountering things like panic attacks and anxiety-inducing situations. But more on that later.

Eat slowly and mindfully

Often we eat our food in such a hurry and with such distraction. We look at it as a secondary task, and if you're anything like me, you like to watch or read something when you eat too. But this seemingly harmless act could actually be doing our digestion a disservice and so it's important to try and be as mindful as possible when eating to get the very most from your digestion.

Try and chew your food as much as possible, eat slowly, don't gulp or take in lots of air between mouthfuls, don't drink fizzy drinks with your food (or if you're like me, at all, as I am just a burping, fizzy, puffy mess if I drink fizzy pop) and enjoy your food. Think about the smell, the taste, the texture. Enjoy your food - fully!

Food diary set-up

As mentioned above, I had a very specific food diary set-up in the initial months of cutting out dairy and eggs that really helped me to figure out what my IBS was reacting to and what my trigger foods were.

Let's go through an example together:

MONDAY

- BREAKFAST:

Porridge with rice milk, a teaspoon of maple syrup

Tummy: I went to the toilet after my porridge and my stomach felt settled

- SNACK:

Banana and two oatcakes

Tummy: It felt settled

- LUNCH:

Avocado and chicken wrap with tomatoes

Tummy: Felt a bit bubbly after lunch but I settled it with a peppermint tea

- DINNER:

Chicken, red peppers, rice and salad leaves

Tummy: Felt settled and relaxed.

I'd then continue this on throughout the week, occasionally reintroducing things to test the reaction, and then monitoring how my stomach felt.

It's an ongoing process and even now, my body reacts differently to things that it used to love or hate - so it can be worth re-testing annually.

If in doubt, stick to soothing foods *(though again, monitor them, in case they do irritate your symptoms)*, such as mint, oats, fennel, bananas, chicken broth, coconut milk, chicken, rice, potatoes, ginger.

I have provided some tummy-friendly recipes towards the end of the book, just in case you need a few fail-safes to get you going.

Above all else, know that it's going to take some time to figure out what works best for you.

Everybody is different and every set of IBS symptoms is also very different, so be kind to yourself, keep a food diary and listen to your body.

IBS-related diets can be very restrictive (and it's important NOT to cut vital food groups out of your diet it's unless absolutely necessary), so my motto when it comes to food now is:

'Eat to make your body happy.'

In the very general sense of the phrase, you should listen to your body and feed it food that makes it the happiest, healthiest and most calm it can be.

Sometimes, I have to live off very plain 'beige' food, such as potatoes, rice, chicken and oats, when I'm suffering from a grumbling tummy.

Other times, I can get a little more adventurous.

I suppose it's all part of the IBS expedition.

But I do believe that having IBS has benefitted me in ways that I didn't initially expect. Whereas other young people my age could arguably be 'punishing' their body with heavy nights out, gallons of fizzy pop and junk food – I've had to learn to fuel my body in the best way possible and be mindful of how everything that I'm putting in affects it.

Some may say it ruins the 'fun', but I think it's a privilege to learn how to do this while I'm still young.

You often hear of many people going through life being able to eat and drink what they'd like, only to have a huge wake-up call when a major health issue presents itself later on down the line.

We have to be quite disciplined early on, but it will pay off in the long run, I truly believe that!

Below I have put together a list of common trigger foods and irritants for IBS sufferers, just to act as a starting point for your initial food diary. Obviously you may not react to some, or indeed even any of them, but they are a good foundation if you're unsure of what to keep an eye on first.

- CAFFEINE

- DAIRY

- EGGS

- GLUTEN

- WHEAT

- ONIONS

- GARLIC

- ALCOHOL

- HIGHLY PROCESSED AND HIGH FAT FOODS

- REFINED SUGAR

- CARBONATED/FIZZY DRINKS

- BEANS

- RED MEAT

- ACIDIC FRUITS

- SUGAR SUBSTITUTES WITHIN 'SUGAR-FREE' FOODS

Usually as a general rule, when I'm having a flare-up, I try not to eat food items bought from the supermarket with ingredients I don't recognise. Take it back to basics and then slowly re-introduce small amounts of certain foods to see how they fare.

Medication is a really tricky subject because the right medication can help some people immensely in regaining their quality of life back and, therefore, it's a necessity.

I also appreciate that doctors are always trying their best to make sure that each patient leaves with something new to try, or a proactive step to combat the symptoms.

CHAPTER 4

Medication

Doctors are so short of time as it is, especially in the UK, so they don't always have the resources to really get to the bottom of a patient's individual symptoms and figure out why they might be occurring.

They are there to listen, give a diagnosis and a prescription.

I spent several years on different medications, but unfortunately found that while the original symptom or complaint may have been temporarily masked by a particular medication, other symptoms would then present themselves in its place.

For example, I'd be prescribed Loperamide for my various toilet trips, only to suffer from serious constipation and angry bowel sounds when I took it. So, yes, I didn't have diarrhoea any longer but I now had a new symptom (or series of symptoms) to tackle.

Nothing really gave me back my equilibrium and got to the root cause of why those symptoms were appearing in the first place.

At one point, my family called me the 'walking pharmacist' because of all the various over-the-counter and prescription medications I was carrying for my IBS symptoms. Different symptoms would present themselves at random intervals, so I prepared myself for every eventuality.

Although some would disappear for a few hours, which was enough to get me through some difficult exams and lectures, they'd usually come back with a vengeance afterwards and I'd have to take a step back.

I still felt my body was out of control, possibly more than ever, as I didn't know what new symptom would present itself after it masked another.

Over the years, I tried mebeverine, laxatives, Imodium, antacid, calcium carbonate, to name just a few.

I also tried beta-blockers and anti-depressants as the symptoms starting affecting my mental health and my ability to complete my studies.

All to no avail.

I felt all the medicine I took masked a symptom I was suffering from. It wasn't getting to the root cause of WHY I was suffering from that particular symptom.

It wasn't determining what my body was reacting to and how I could really fix it.

I suppose it's very much like a house. You might keep getting cracks, or damp marks on the ceiling or water leaks. Sure, you could keep patching up those issues without spending too much time or money. But you haven't got to the root cause of why you're getting water leaks. So they keep popping back up and you have to keep putting the house back together. But once you find the source of what's causing the issues and fix that, all of the issues disappear.

Later in the book, I go into detail about the other causes of your symptoms. While I definitely cannot diagnose you (and even Dr Google can't either, please visit your GP), it is really interesting to know that there could be other reasons for some of your symptoms. Everything is worth researching into because the more you know, the closer you may get to figuring out WHY those symptoms are happening in the first place. And don't just trust one article, read around the subject. If you have the time (and inclination) read medical journals, read books and read magazine articles. It will all help you to understand your situation, your body, your mind, your symptoms and how each of those things reacts with your IBS.

Anyway, back to medication.

Medicine is a very personal thing and I'm certainly not here to bash it entirely.

In fact, if you have indeed found a medication that really helps with your symptoms, then that is great news and a huge relief for you!

But if you can try to manage your symptoms through your diet, therapy and natural supplements (which we will talk about later), then it's certainly worth looking into. I am so much happier, healthier and less affected by my symptoms since choosing to do this myself.

I found my solutions through natural remedies and got to the bottom of tackling the root cause of each symptom. It often takes longer to see the results as they're not synthetic chemicals and formulations, but a far more long-term solution that helps you to become (and to stay) in tune with your body.

I'd thoroughly recommend you see a good, reputable nutritionist to get a personalised list of what supplements you should be taking. I started seeing one almost a year ago now, and while it's certainly not cheap, I've learned so much about my body and healed it from the inside.

Again, it's a very personal decision as to what avenue you choose to go down, but I've personally found an immense amount of help and advice from the results produced by this machine. I started visiting them on the personal recommendation of a friend after she recovered from a similar chronic condition.

I've written an entire chapter further on in the book regarding supplements and natural remedies, so I won't go into any further depth here, but to finish, I just want to add a few things that my doctors were invaluable for along my IBS journey.

TESTS

In order to eliminate any further worry or anxiety about your symptoms, I'd recommend requesting as many formal tests through your doctor as you can.

I went through a period of feeling very anxious that the severity of my symptoms might mean that they were a result of another, life-threatening condition.

A simple Google search of your symptoms can quickly spiral into thoughts like, 'Oh my goodness, could it be this or this,' followed morbidly by, 'I must be dying'.

When I was at university and suffering my most severe symptoms, I was convinced that the agonising pain was the result of something far more sinister.

I lay awake at night worrying about whether I was in the midst of a terrible illness and Dr Google kept presenting the C word. It's commonly known that IBS symptoms can be rather similar to the largely invisible ovarian cancer. Which is why I cannot emphasise enough how important it is to visit your doctor for the reassurance you need - as well of course, to rule out any underlying conditions.

Often I speak to other sufferers who have been too scared to visit their doctors, afraid they will have to undergo humiliating examinations or invasive tests without prior warning. Many people also resist visiting their doctors for fear of 'making a fuss over nothing' or not wanting to cause a fuss. However, I would implore you to seek professional advice and if you and your doctor deem it necessary, eliminate further worry by undergoing as many formal tests as you/they see fit.

In the initial stages of investigating my symptoms, I was absolutely terrified I was going to visit the doctor only for them to ask me to lay on the bed to 'inspect' my bottom. But rest assured, doctors are there to make you feel comfortable, to be an ear to listen to your concerns and to assist in coming up with solutions to make you better. They see patients on a daily basis with a variety of ailments and so there is no need to ever feel self-conscious.

I personally haven't ever experienced any kind of embarrassment during a doctors appointment. Usually an initial consultation involves answering questions about your bowel movements (one quiz I don't need to revise for), a little prod of the tummy and a referral for a blood test.

In the end, my parents frogmarched me to the doctors and demanded I undergo as many tests as I could to determine what on earth was going on.

I underwent blood tests, ultrasounds, and later down the line, had a colonoscopy.

The latter of which was extremely reassuring, as I could, quite literally, see my insides – with my very own eyes –on a screen in front of me.

For those of you who are fortunate enough NOT to know what a colonoscopy procedure is, it essentially involves a doctor putting a very small camera up your bottom and then through your large bowel and intestines.

It's not the most pleasant of experiences as you can imagine, but you can ask to be sedated so that you're very relaxed.

And of course, it's something that is booked in advance and conducted in a hospital - so you have plenty of time to prepare.

My favourite part of the colonoscopy ordeal is the prep, which involves taking a wonderful water-based solution called Moviprep in the 24 hours leading up to your procedure.

Essentially, it empties you from the inside out and clears your 'system' ready for inspection.

Things start off slowly before gathering momentum until you're pretty much peeing out of your bum.

It's all very painless and as long as you're in the comfort of your own home, absolutely fine.

But I would recommend stocking up on wet wipes and a lined bin, which you should strategically place in your bathroom. Otherwise, you're at risk of blocking up your toilet with tissue paper. I may or may not be speaking from experience.

Afterwards, you feel very EMPTY, for lack of a better word. It's quite a nice feeling, especially if you're usually prone to constipation and constantly feeling blocked up and bloated.

I wasn't lying when I said it was my favourite part.

The next day, you visit the hospital (nil by mouth for 12 hours previously), pop on your fancy hospital gown (I like to think of them of boho-chic, with a backwards wrap dress design - that exposes your bottom - *fabulous*) and lay down on the bed, on your side.

I'll be honest, the sedation kicked in pretty quickly and I don't remember the camera 'going in'.

However, the doctor struggled quite a bit with my colonoscopy, as he discovered that I have a much longer, loopier bowel than normal with many twists and turns in it.

When trying to put the camera through my intestines, it would scrape against the sides or get stuck trying to manoeuvre around a corner. I'm not going to sugar coat the experience and say it was fine because it was blooming painful. However I do think that this was in part due to my colon being longer and more twisty than your average one. Many people I've spoken with who have also had a colonoscopy had a very painless experience, with just a slight bit of discomfort.

Luckily, throughout I had a lovely nurse alongside me, who squeezed my hand, stroked my head and gave me gas and air for pain relief when it all got a bit too much. It really did make all the difference and in my sedated, woozy state - I didn't thank her properly for being so kind and comforting. It really did make the world of difference.

Thankfully, the doctors didn't find anything untoward, although they did take a few biopsies (which I saw him taking on the screen – watching someone cut bits out of you in front of your eyes makes you feel extremely mortal) just to be sure.

But the relief I felt afterwards, knowing that I'd been investigated thoroughly and taken seriously, was well worth the pain and discomfort the colonoscopy caused.

It also helped me to understand my digestive system, as the 'longer and loopier' characteristic of my colon was an explanation for why I had a longer transit time than usual and why dairy is such a big trigger in causing abdominal pain for me - as it gets stuck in the 'loops', the sugars ferment as they are attempted to be broken down and this invariably causes issues.

Again, it's all about feeling in tune with your body, and this particular procedure really helped to reassure me by calming the anxious part of my brain which, in turn, helped with my IBS in general.

Things to consider

○ HAVE YOU VISITED YOUR GP TO EXPLAIN YOUR SYMPTOMS AND/OR ANY ANXIETY SURROUNDING THOSE SYMPTOMS?

○ HAVE YOU UNDERGONE THE NECESSARY TESTS TO ENSURE IT ISN'T ANYTHING OTHER THAN IBS OR DIGESTIVE DISCOMFORT?

○ HAVE YOU MADE NOTE OF YOUR MOST BOTHERSOME SYMPTOMS?

○ HAVE YOU FOUND ANY MEDICATIONS THAT TOTALLY RELIEVE YOU OF YOUR SYMPTOMS?

○ HAVE YOU DONE YOUR OWN RESEARCH INTO OTHER REMEDIES FOR YOUR SYMPTOMS?

○ ARE YOU INTERESTED IN SEEING IF NATURAL SUPPLEMENTS COULD HELP PROVIDE SOME RELIEF FROM YOUR SYMPTOMS?

SUPPLEMENTS

There are SO many supplements on the market that claim to help with IBS-related digestive symptoms and while I'm sure many of them CAN be helpful in their own individual way, it's a bit of a minefield when it comes to figuring out where on earth to start.

Again, it's all about research (sorry to sound like a broken record), since what works for one person, may not for another.

Often some IBS symptoms are the result of a mineral or vitamin deficiency.

For example, boosting your magnesium intake can be very beneficial for IBS sufferers who are prone to constipation. It has also been proven to help with anxiety, taking the edge off and easing a low mood. However, it might also not help at all. Like all of the above, it's a case of trial and error. There's no one-size-fits-all method.

My overriding advice would be to do thorough research or consult a nutritionist or specialist.

I wholeheartedly believe that even if you have an absolutely PERFECT diet, you could benefit from certain supplements because there are many vitamins and minerals our bodies might not digest properly. For example, my body lacked iron. Although I was eating plenty of leafy greens, it wasn't being absorbed because I had other deficiencies too.

I have found immense relief after trialling a variety of supplements and I believe that an effective management plan for IBS does involve a couple of different ones, especially at the beginning.

Obviously, they're not the same as medication, so you're not going to get immediate relief. I think the benefits of supplements are often widely underestimated because of this. You do have to be patient and make sure that you are providing the best possible foundations (in other areas of IBS management) to ensure they do their job as best they can. But used in the right way, you can really start to see some results after 3-4 weeks. Sometimes sooner.

Supplements can start getting quite expensive and overwhelming, so rather than forking out hundreds of pounds on supplements that you're not sure will work, I'd start with the foundations...

PROBIOTICS

Probiotic is pretty much a buzzword of the last few years. You can now buy probiotic yoghurt, chocolate and even drinks. They seem to be everywhere but does anyone actually know what they do? Can IBS sufferers really benefit or are they just a scheme to make money? And if they are helpful, there's SO many out there. So how do I know which one is right for me?

Good question! First things first, let's talk about bacteria. As much as we've grown up thinking 'bacteria' is always a bad thing, our bodies actually contain millions of good bacteria, which help to keep your gut nice and healthy. Because the majority of our immune system resides within the gut, beneficial bacteria help to support your body's natural defences. Our gut flora (the hive of good bacteria) helps protect us against getting poorly, it maintains a kind of 'equilibrium' and a harmonious space inside us. It aids healthy digestion, skin, and overall health.

When we take antibiotics, to fight off infection, it heads to the gut and kills off ALL the bacteria, as it's not quite clever enough to differentiate between the 'good' bacteria (i.e. the little friendly guys that help to keep us healthy) and the 'bad' bacteria (that make us ill and cause us to take the antibiotics in the first place). This is why a lot of people develop IBS like symptoms after a bout of illness or food poisoning. Because they have a lack of good bacteria in the gut and there's no longer digestive harmony. Medication can upset the equilibrium.

However even if you haven't taken antibiotics, gut bacteria can also be unbalanced due to diet (even if you have a healthy intake, these fussy bacteria need a DIVERSE diet to thrive and survive), drinking too much alcohol, smoking and even not getting enough sleep.

You can read more about probiotics and their benefits but essentially, they help to restore our gut flora which can, in turn, restore our digestive 'normality'. When I first started taking probiotics aged 19, I found they helped to reset my gut and take the edge off my symptoms.

For some people, their symptoms can worsen in the initial stages, especially if there's a lot of work for the probiotics to do. Usually, this means it's getting to work resetting things, which is a good sign. But it's also the common reason why most people give up on them and don't stick with them. It usually takes 9-12 weeks to notice a considerable difference and for your gut flora to be reset.

I now take probiotics daily and since doing so, I am pleased to say I've not only achieved digestive harmony, but I've also reaped the benefits of them boosting my immune system too. I haven't had a 'cold' or the flu in over three years (and counting). And this is coming from a girl who ALWAYS used to be off sick for catching whatever bug was going round. If I am ever ill with a snotty nose or cough, it's usually out of me within 24 hours and does not knock me out like it used to.

My skin also improved and cleared up in the same time frame, which was another huge bonus! I often find building up your good bacteria can also take the edge off any food triggers. Obviously, this won't be relevant for everyone, but since I started taking probiotics daily, I don't have as much of a drastic a reaction if any dairy has snuck into my food. A special thanks to one restaurant who helped me test out this hypothesis. They insisted no dairy was present, only to later tell me 'there was cheese in the sauce, but it was cooked, so surely that would have been okay?' Err nope, cooked or not, dairy is dairy.

For any IBS sufferer, weaving in a daily probiotic should be a staple - and as with anything, if the first one doesn't work for you, don't be put off - try another. Different brands and products contain different strains of good bacteria - and eventually, one will fit with you.

Some probiotics are kept in the fridge, others are in liquid form and others can be stored in the cupboard - so also be sure to check the instructions on how to store and take them. Usually they are to be taken before food or first thing in the morning. This can make a big difference in how effective they are.

I currently use a range of different probiotics which have each helped me at different stages of my IBS recovery journey. Symprove was an amazing starting point for me, as it's a liquid solution that heads straight to the gut and gets to work populating your gut with good bacteria that survive and thrive. I initially found my symptoms worsened in the first week, but I'm glad I persevered because they soon improved and took the edge off my abdominal pain and soothed my digestion, resulting in far less toilet trips. Symprove is kept in the fridge and taken first thing in the morning, 10 minutes before food. They have a wonderful customer service team who were on hand to answer any questions and generally support me when I was going through a tough time during a flare up of symptoms.

On a daily basis and while I am travelling, I use Alflorex and Just For Tummies Live Bacteria - as I've experienced success with both. Alflorex was something I used during a really tough time a few years ago when my stomach was very upset and very vocal. It really calmed my stomach 'noises' and put me back on track.

Just For Tummies is another product I use on a daily basis to promote general harmony within my digestive system and keep it calm while travelling (I took it with me on a week long camping trip recently and it helped me manage - despite a new routine and time zone.

As I mentioned above, each probiotic is unique and different things work for different people. So don't be put off if your first experience wasn't successful. Again, it's worth keeping track of how you feel while taking a new supplement to attribute any improvements.

It usually takes between six and twelve weeks to 'reset' your gut bacteria, so it is worth persevering.

I am of the opinion that a 'diverse and varied' gut bacteria is only a good thing, so I am on a mission to support this within my own body as much as I can, using foods, probiotics and a healthy lifestyle!

Activated Charcoal

It sounds like a very odd thing to put into your body, but activated charcoal can be a huge help to those of you who find that wind, gas and bloating is a massive issue.

Activated charcoal can gently absorb bubbles of uncomfortable gas, helping to expel them more discreetly.

There are also 'activated charcoal' biscuits available from health food shops that I used to take into exams/lessons with me and munch on to calm my stomach. However, if you are sensitive to dairy, be aware some of them may contain butter.

Please make sure you consult your doctor before using any supplements.

Aloe Vera

If you, like me, are prone to constipation but you've found that traditional remedies send you the other way, then I'd opt for weaving in some Aloe Vera into your daily routine, as a means of combating this. Aloe Vera is a natural supplement that has anti-inflammatory and slight laxative effects. So it soothes your system and keeps you regular. A win-win!

Aloe Vera juice helps digestion, normalises acid/alkaline and pH balance, lessens yeast formation, encourages digestive bacteria and regularises bowel processing, so it's fabulous for a whole host of digestive issues.

You can take Aloe Vera in several different formats and the one you go for depends on your daily routine and whether you like the taste.

Capsule forms are available in your local health food shop and can be really effective. However, I find I get the most benefit from the drink forms, as you can almost feel the soothing effects instantly wash through your digestive system and get things moving quickly.

The liquid food supplements usually need to be kept in the fridge and a small dose is taken each morning. I did this for a little while, but it got a bit tricky when I was travelling, so I also buy Simplee Aloe with White Grape Juice drink, which I have with my breakfast and can take around in a little carton.

Again, this all depends on you personally, so it's worth a little bit of trial and error to make sure you figure out which one works best for you.

Other supplements commonly associated with easing IBS symptoms include:

O   MILK THISTLE

O   CHAMOMILE

O   PEPPERMINT

O   LIQUORICE

O   CBD OIL

O   BETAINE HYDROCHLORIDE WITH PEPSIN

O   BLACKSTRAP MOLASSES

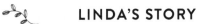

Linda Booth is a leading natural digestive health expert with 26 years' experience of running a natural health clinic, specialising in solutions to resolve common digestive and gut disorders, such as Irritable Bowel Syndrome (IBS), painful bloating, constipation, diarrhoea, heartburn and indigestion. I have been in touch with Linda for the past few years and she has very kindly been there for me on email and in person to provide heartfelt and practical advice for managing and controlling my symptoms. She knows IBS inside and out and has a plethora of helpful resources on her website, Just For Tummies, which also happens to be the hub of her supplement company, of the same name.

I've been taking Linda's probiotics daily for the last year and have found them immensely helpful in keeping my stomach balanced and giving it an equilibrium. She kindly agreed to chat with me and have our conversation published in this book. For more specific and tailored advice from Linda, it's worth reaching out to her individually as she's always happy to give helpful advice, depending on your symptoms.

How beneficial do you think supplements are for the treatment of IBS?

Supplements, particularly live bacteria probiotics and digestive enzymes, are crucial in the successful management of IBS, and if you're not eating oily fish at least twice weekly, a high-strength Omega 3 fish oil capsule too.

How do IBS sufferers successfully manage their condition? Is it something we will always have to suffer from?

Firstly, IBS sufferers need to understand why they have IBS in the first place. I'm passionate about education and awareness of the causes of IBS. I don't like to be a pessimist as I'm very much a 'glass half full girl', but until people understand the impact that their diets and lifestyles have on their digestive and gut health, together with the impact that stress and medications have, we will see more and more people diagnosed with this debilitating condition.

Anyone that suspects they have IBS must firstly go and see their GP. Certain conditions need to be excluded, including Coeliac disease, inflammatory bowel diseases, like Crohn's disease, and ulcerative colitis, as well as ovarian cancer and bowel cancer. Once the GP has ruled out all the aforementioned, the diagnosis is usually one of IBS.

In your experience of treating many IBS patients, are there any 'hidden' symptoms that are not usually associated with IBS you see a lot of?

With IBS, there is an imbalance in the gut microbiome, with the potential to cause low-grade inflammation in the small intestine. This can affect absorption of nutrients, leading to fatigue, weight gain, hormonal imbalances, depression, anxiety, skin problems and an increased risk of auto-immune diseases. Remember that around 80% of your immune cells are manufactured in your small intestine. If your small intestine is irritated and inflamed, this can weaken your immune system, making you less resilient to infections and diseases.

How can an IBS sufferer prevent excess gas?

Always chew each mouthful at least 20 times and don't eat when feeling stressed, angry or anxious. Don't eat too much, too fast or too late. Take a digestive enzyme to help digest protein with carbs and try to eat low FODMAP vegetables, like potatoes, carrots, bean sprouts. Get the Monash University FODMAP diet app. It tells you all you need to know about FODMAP and what to eat and what not to eat. Impaction in the bowel can create lots of 'toxic' gases, causing painful bloating, so eat enough fibre to avoid constipation and stay hydrated.

Are there any 'quick fixes' or tips to eliminating or minimising bloating?

All IBS sufferers should be taking a live bacteria probiotic capsule before breakfast and one before bed to help heal the gut and minimise gas production and bloating. You can also take 2/3 charcoal capsules half an hour before meals. Charcoal helps to absorb trapped painful gases.

What are your most popular supplements?

My 'bestsellers' are my Live Bacteria probiotic capsules, my Digestive Enzyme tablets, my For Women probiotic capsules and my Charcoal capsules. All made in the UK, vegan and gluten-free.

How would someone weave in supplements into their daily routine?

Always keep your supplements where you can see them. Don't stick them in a drawer or cupboard where they will be forgotten. If you want to put them in a drawer, put them in the cutlery drawer. We go in the cutlery drawer several times a day, so we don't forget to take our supplements. All my supplements contain dosage information on the back label, but people are also welcome to contact me direct for more specific advice. With supplements, the key is getting into a routine with them, a bit like cleaning your teeth. Once you get into a routine, it's easy. It's also a good idea to keep a pot of the supplements at work.

I think a three-pronged treatment approach to IBS worked best for me – diet, therapy and supplements. Would you agree and do you have any additional things to add?

Each case of IBS is different. Our gut microbiome is as unique as our fingerprint, and what works for one person may not be as successful for another. However, without a shadow of a doubt, probiotics, digestive enzymes and attention to healthy eating have always improved symptoms. Hypnotherapy, meditation and mindfulness are recommended in those people whose IBS flares up during a stressful period, so I absolutely agree, Scarlett, it has to be a multi-pronged approach for the best outcome.

Are you able to briefly explain the benefit of 'good bacteria' from probiotics and why an IBS patient might find a huge improvement from implementing them into their daily routine?

I've been in practice for 27 years and carried out over 80,000 consultations and treatments and every IBS patient who has attended my clinic has found an improvement in their symptoms after taking a course of my Live Bacteria probiotic capsules. The gut of an IBS suffer is out of balance and, in many cases, also inflamed. Probiotics also help to digest food, absorb nutrients, help to 'crowd' out pathogenic strains of bacteria, as well as positively influence our immune system, making us more resilient to infections. Probiotics help to recolonise and replenish the gut, calming down inflammation, reducing gas and reducing bloating and pain. Certain species of probiotics are more effective than others, which is why my Live Bacteria contain Lactobacillus acidophilus and Lactobacillus rhamnosus, two strains proven to reduce bloating and abdominal pain.

As IBS is just an umbrella term for a collection of symptoms, would you say that symptoms COULD also be caused by other things, such as SIBO, Leaky Gut etc? If so, what can you tell me about these things?

If someone is a chronic IBS sufferer, then there is a good chance that they may have 'leaky' gut and small intestinal bacterial overgrowth (SIBO) as well. However, to positively confirm these conditions, it requires a stool test. Again, our gut microbiome is as unique as our fingerprint, so one person may suffer from IBS and the next may have IBS, SIBO and 'leaky' gut. It all depends upon what their digestive system and gut have been exposed to over the years, how strong their immune system is and their constitution. The typical symptom of SIBO is bloating on waking, and typical symptoms of 'leaky' gut are headaches and fatigue, but it is not black and white. They may also want to consider having a test for parasites.

What advice would you give to someone who is at their wit's end with their symptoms and doesn't even know where to start on the road to recovery?

If someone is at their wit's end, I would encourage them to talk to someone. Don't be embarrassed about their IBS. Around 20% of the UK population suffer from IBS so that's over 12 million people. They are not on their own. It's important to get help to ensure that the IBS symptoms are not a red herring, and it's nothing more serious that is causing the symptoms. They can join my Tummy Talk Facebook community, that I monitor. I have many complementary medicine practitioners in Tummy Talk, who are all very experienced in treating people who have IBS, or they can just drop me an email and I will help. If I can't help, I signpost them to someone who can. They can also consider seeking the advice of a registered and regulated nutritional therapist. There's lots of advice about what people with IBS should and shouldn't do and much of it is poor quality, leading people down a path that exacerbates their IBS.

EACH CASE OF IBS IS DIFFERENT.

OUR GUT MICROBIOME IS AS UNIQUE AS

OUR FINGERPRINT AND WHAT WORKS FOR

ONE PERSON, MAY NOT BE AS

SUCCESSFUL FOR ANOTHER.

Although most people have now heard of the term IBS, many people don't know it is actually a very broad term that encompasses a whole host of symptoms. Often 'Irritable Bowel' is presented as a 'diagnosis' after several other conditions have been eliminated.

CHAPTER 5

What else could it be?

BS is an umbrella term used to describe a series of symptoms with no dedicated pattern, cure or one single trigger (i.e. a virus, contagion or stimulant). This makes it extremely difficult to treat and means that it is really a case of 'trial and error' for each individual as a means of figuring out what makes YOUR body tick.

For years, I wasn't quite ready (or perhaps willing) to dedicate the amount of time needed to research what is a very complex condition. It's a complete minefield and totally overwhelming when you're already exhaustingly having to navigate your life with a series of symptoms that are hell-bent on making things very difficult for you.

However, a very nasty flare-up in 2015 encouraged me to pause and reflect, as I was spending an awful lot of time practically bedbound in pain (between various bathroom visits) and I had the time and inclination to really research the individual symptoms and WHY they might each be occurring.

As I've mentioned before, I'm definitely not a doctor, medical expert or health practitioner – this is just my journey of discovering the causes of each of my symptoms and working out ways to understand them better.

I soon discovered there are SO many related conditions to IBS that often have a greater understanding and they provide a more helpful path to potential recovery. I'll go through each of these conditions and then, at the end, chat about how you could go about testing for these conditions and the next steps you can look into.

I can't empathise enough how daunting it might seem initially, but the more knowledge we equip ourselves with, the more likely we are to find out a management plan that gives us back control. It's important to stay positive (as hard as that can be) and envision yourself getting better, as the mind is a very powerful tool that drives us forward so that we stay on track and achieve what we want to.

I lost hope for a long time, but finally regained it when I imagined exactly what it was that I wanted to get out of my life at that point in time, which was my journalism degree. It was so important to me to power on and know in my heart that I WAS going to find a solution.

LEAKY GUT

The inside of our bowels are lined by a single layer of cells called the mucosal barrier, which is a very effective part of our digestive system that absorbs nutrients and prevents large molecules of food and bacteria from crossing over and passing into our bloodstream.

Leaky gut is potentially a pretty common condition in the Western world and it refers to increased intestinal permeability – in other words, toxins and the food we consume. Bacteria is able to 'leak' through the intestinal wall before being flagged up as an 'intruder' within our bloodstream, causing a whole host of issues, such as food intolerances, digestive irritability and sensitivity and other IBS-related symptoms.

This condition hasn't been recognised formally (especially in the UK); however, research and information online are gathering momentum, and it has been linked to a whole host of long-term issues, such as MS and chronic fatigue syndrome. According to the NHS, common contributors and causes for a potential 'leaky gut' can include bowel lining irritants, such as Ibuprofen, aspirin and even alcohol.

Exponents of Leaky Gut syndrome (who are mostly alternative therapy practitioners and nutritionists) have also claimed that the prevalence of antibiotics in modern society may also be to blame for a 'widespread Leaky Gut' problem, as they get rid of the good bacteria in the gut that provide vital protection against this happening.

Many believe that Leaky Gut can be 'reset' by following a low FODMAP diet, taking a good probiotic daily and other supplements that promote healthy fungal levels in the bowel (such as Caprin).

If you suspect that your symptoms may be the result of Leaky Gut, it would worth consulting your health practitioner. There is no specific testing within general medicine that can be conducted to flag this particular condition, but it's worth doing some research into this yourself and looking into seeing an alternative medicine practitioner. I was tested for Leaky Gut with a SCIO machine by a natural health therapist, and after taking supplements, I found my associated symptoms got much better.

I'm sure any IBS sufferer (or chronic illness patient) can understand we'll try anything once if there's a chance of us getting better or getting relief from our symptoms. Everyone will be different and some people may be cynical (I totally understand this and it's your right to have a difference in opinion on this), but I personally found real relief from my symptoms after being treated for Leaky Gut.

SIBO

Small intestinal bacterial overgrowth (SIBO) is a condition affecting the small intestine.

It occurs when bacteria that normally grows in other parts of the gut begin growing in the small intestine, eventually causing pain, diarrhoea and severe bloating. It can also begin to use up the bodies nutrients and therefore cause malnutrition and malabsorption.

Some believe that SIBO is caused by a bout of stomach flu, virus or gastroenteritis (food poisoning); however, as with Leaky Gut, it is still pretty under-researched in the UK (although I do believe it is more widely spoken about in the US as a specific condition and diagnosis).

Unlike the conditions above, there is a formal test for the presence of SIBO in the form of a breath test. Excess bacteria in the small intestine can lead to the release of the gases hydrogen and methane, which can be identified through a breath test. This test is non-invasive and can be performed at home or at your doctor's. If you suspect that you may have this, it is worth asking your doctor for advice on the next steps, although testing may have to be done privately rather than on the NHS.

Probiotics and a special diet can provide some relief for the symptoms associated with SIBO; however, of course, it's worth consulting your health practitioner on their opinion before self-diagnosing or using any supplements.

BAD

IBS is invariably going to be different for everyone, and the trial and error rollercoaster of what works for you – gluten-free, dairy-free, wheat-free, CBT etc. – can feel a little exhausting.

If nothing still seems to be working, you may be suffering from something called BAD or Bile Acid Diarrhoea (another sympathetic term, I'm sure you'll agree).

Symptomised by chronic diarrhoea, BAD is thought to have over 1,000,000 sufferers in the UK and is, thankfully, quite treatable. In fact, one in three people who are diagnosed with IBS will actually have BAD.

Symptoms of BAD can vary from person to person. There is often a long history of chronic diarrhoea that is often diagnosed as severe IBS. Many people have the symptoms for many years, some in excess of a decade. The most common symptoms of BAD are painful, watery, explosive chronic diarrhoea, urgently needing the toilet/having accidents, numerous bowel movements a day that often occur during the night, foul-smelling diarrhoea which is yellow/greasy in appearance, excessive wind, painful stomach cramps and moderate to severe bloating.

There are currently different tests available to help reach a diagnosis of BAD and some of these tests are blood tests which measure different biomarkers. There is also a scan which is non-invasive and involves swallowing a capsule containing synthetic bile acids.

Bile Acid Sequestrants (BAS) are usually prescribed to help manage the symptoms of bile acid diarrhoea. The medications work by binding to the bile acids in the small bowel and preventing them from irritating the large intestine. It may take several days before an improvement in the diarrhoea is seen and several weeks or months to find the right level of medication and dietary adaptation that help to control the symptoms.

Once a diagnosis of bile acid diarrhoea is made it is advisable to see a doctor and a dietician, since a key piece of dietary advice may be to follow a low-fat diet. There are other specialised diets that can be recommended and your dietician will be able to go through these in far more detail.

PARASITE

I used to think that having a 'worm' inside you was a myth until it happened to me, and I actually saw the said creature when I went to the toilet. I wish I was joking and I'm so sorry we've entered another level of TMI here. I've really been through the wringer with all these various digestive conditions and, unfortunately, I can add 'parasite' to this seemingly never-ending list.

Having a 'parasite' can be an extremely daunting and pretty terrifying thought, but it's far more common than you think and it CAN cause some of the digestive symptoms commonly associated with IBS too. Thankfully, they are treatable. However, like me, you may find that you have been blessed with a parasite, as well as general IBS.

Parasites can cause symptoms such as:

O   BLOATING

O   DIARRHOEA

O   FATIGUE OR WEAKNESS

O   GAS

O   NAUSEA

O   STOMACH PAIN OR TENDERNESS

O   VOMITING

O   ITCHING AROUND THE BOTTOM

O   TROUBLE FALLING ASLEEP OR IRRITABILITY AT NIGHT

O   TEETH GRINDING

- O NEVER QUITE FEELING FULL OR SATISFIED AFTER A MEAL

- O UNEXPLAINED SKIN IRRITATIONS, RASHES AND HIVES

You have a history of food poisoning and your digestion hasn't been the same since

And then the most fabulous one of all, actually passing a worm in your stool. I thought I was hallucinating. I wondered if I needed glasses. I couldn't quite believe it. It was teeny tiny but sure enough, very real. Then, after being diagnosed, I felt deeply, hideously ashamed of myself – all at the same time.

Essentially, a parasite is an organism that lives and feeds off a host.

So an internal parasite in the digestive system is a worm (or worms) that feed off your nutrition.

Some examples of parasites include pinworms, roundworms, hookworms, and tapeworms. Don't ask me the difference between them and maybe don't Google them either. I wouldn't recommend it. The results are pretty graphic and will probably put you right off your next meal.

Unfortunately, because parasites vary so much in shape and size, they can create a wide range of different issues.

If you have unexplained weight loss, you are unable to gain weight or you're still hungry after each meal, you may find that you have a parasite consuming your food.

Some may feed off of your red blood cells, causing symptoms of anaemia such as fatigue, shortness of breath and a lack of energy.

Others parasites lay eggs that can trigger irritation, itching, and sleeping problems such as insomnia.

If you have tried and tested many approaches in a bid to alleviate your symptoms and soothe your gut without any relief, a parasite might just be the concealed cause.

There is definitely a HUGE stigma attached to parasites and they are very, very rarely spoken about. However, it may be worth getting tested for one because they can usually be easily treated at your doctors.

I was prescribed medication and they went away. I've thankfully never had another bout of them, but prevention revolves around practising good hygiene levels and washing your hands frequently. Sometimes. parasites can be contracted through the food you eat (meat, salads etc) or the water you drink. So, when travelling, you should always be aware of what you're eating in respect of where you are. In rare cases, it has even been reported that parasites can enter your body from the bottom of your feet. But don't quote me on that one. Or maybe just wear shoes.

So although there is a stigma attached to parasites, contracting one doesn't necessarily mean that you've been dirty or unhygienic. Even fruits and vegetables can sometimes harbour parasites. However, once you have one, you can very easily pass it on by touching door handles, taps, towels etc, which is why good hygiene thereafter is vital.

As with any new symptoms or issues, you should obviously visit your GP to conduct further investigations and look into what could be causing you issues, but I found that doing lots of research myself (and then putting my findings to my GP) was very helpful in tackling my symptoms and finding a tailor-made solution.

A SENSITIVE STOMACH

As it's widely understood to be the 'second brain' in our bodies, our gut – or stomach area – is understandably going to be affected by external stressors.

The term 'butterflies in your stomach' applies whenever you feel anxious or nervous and is usually a positive thing, as it means you are excited and getting a buzz about something. It's that buzz that drives us forward to do our best job in many instances. However, an overcrowding of butterflies and too much anxious energy can cause a sensitive stomach to go into overdrive. This will produce too much adrenaline unnecessarily which manifests into more worry and more digestive discomfort (aka, a bubbling tummy) because it isn't burned up.

I know that I naturally have a sensitive stomach. I'm a worrier by nature and whenever something is going on in my life, my stomach is the first place to take a hit. So it's all about being aware of this and making sure to give it extra kindness and love whenever you can. This includes getting the right amount of sleep, feeding it the right food and practising mindfulness techniques to relax the mind which, in turn, will relax the stomach. Often these things can be easier said (or written down) than done, but with a bit of practice, you'll be astounded by the difference that exercising your mind can have on your sensitive stomach.

IT'S IMPORTANT TO STAY POSITIVE (AS
HARD AS THAT CAN BE) AND ENVISION
YOURSELF GETTING BETTER, AS THE MIND
IS A VERY POWERFUL TOOL THAT DRIVES
US FORWARD SO THAT WE STAY ON TRACK
AND ACHIEVE WHAT WE WANT TO.

My IBS has seen me through years of school, exams and the beginnings of my work life, so I've certainly experienced first-hand how digestive symptoms can disrupt and play havoc with building a career or trying to 'get the grades'.

CHAPTER 6

Career & Education

There were many occasions where I thought I might have to quit a job or a university course because my IBS had been causing me so many issues.

And I know I'm not alone in this.

When I shared my story with IBS online, my inbox starting filling with messages from people all around the globe who were struggling to hold down a job or complete their exams due to their symptoms.

When partnered with a difficult boss or a not-very-understanding teacher, digestive symptoms can increase twofold.

Because, as we've discussed before, stress can cause a flare-up or worsen your IBS.

But if I'm living proof of anything, it's that you can and will succeed, despite your Irritable Bowel Syndrome. It's not going to hold you back if you don't let it.

Very early on, I took on the mindset that I was never going to let my IBS hold me back. I was never going to let it stop me from achieving my dreams. In fact, I used it to will me on towards those dreams. I used it to motivate me, and to this day, I still maintain this motive.

When I was initially diagnosed, aged 14, I was attending a mixed state secondary school in Hertfordshire. They were very exam result oriented and used to begin each morning assembly with 'X number of days until your exams'. Each morning, as this announcement was made, I could feel my tummy grumbling and bubbling with anxiety.

But luckily for me, they also had a fantastic pastoral care team who always took me and my symptoms seriously. They made arrangements for me to feel as comfortable as possible during my school years and I am so thankful for this.

I sat down with the head of year, presented a doctor's note to them (I would always advise getting a doctor's note in case you need to show it) and we figured out together what arrangements might need to be made.

My main concern was that my symptoms could affect my ability to sit exams. I'd done a couple in the classroom the previous term and it had been hell on earth for me, as I was sitting in silence, in a nightmare situation (with all my peers around me, judging me, or so I had convinced myself) trying to focus on the exam questions, while all I could think about was whether anyone could hear my loud stomach or whether I'd draw attention to myself by running out halfway through to go to the toilet.

So my school made arrangements for me to sit all of my exams in a totally separate room, which put me at complete ease. The private exam room was situated right next to a toilet, so that I could run out if I needed to, and there was usually only one invigilator in the room with me, so I could relax and just focus on the exam in hand.

They also allowed me to bring in a small snack and mug of peppermint tea into my exam room with me. This was especially helpful during the longer exams (2 hours+) when I needed to keep the grumbles at bay. It also meant I could eat little and often to stop the wind and gas building up.

I am very grateful that my school was so accommodating because I know so many of you struggle with being at school and dealing with IBS symptoms. I do think it's worth finding out who is the best person to speak to at your school and setting up a meeting, as the overwhelming sense of relief I felt after putting these arrangements in place was enough to settle my symptoms for a few days.

It's also the reason why I was able to focus solely on working hard and doing the best I possibly could at school. My IBS motivated me to keep pushing on, eager not to be held back. And I'm delighted to say that I left school with 13 A*-B's at GCSE and 2 A's and 2 B's at A Level. I've never been a naturally clever person, who can pass exams effortlessly, but I do work hard and I am so proud that I didn't let my IBS take that away from me.

You can and will succeed despite your symptoms - whether that's exam related, or in other aspects of work. Just make sure that you have the necessary arrangements in place to let your strengths, talents and hard work shine! Help is out there, you just have to ask for it. And if they don't grant you the help you need the first time around, ask someone else!

After finishing school, I decided I wasn't quite ready for university yet, so I deferred my place and got a job at a travel company, in their PR department for the duration of my 'gap year'.

During the first couple of months of working life, I had no symptoms whatsoever. As I was going through an extended symptom-free period, I was able to settle into the 9-5 office job life quite well.

But after a heavy Christmas (I'm looking at you as the main culprit, *Pigs in Blankets*), I returned to the office with my angry symptoms rearing their ugly heads once again. Suddenly, the job I loved was a daily struggle.

My symptoms were not pleasant (six toilet trips each morning, a constantly bubbly gassy stomach and severe pain). This made things like sitting in meetings or being hunched over my desk all day seem near impossible. To anyone else, they were just normal aspects of daily work life. But for me, they were agony. I dreaded them. Feared them.

I remember one particularly unpleasant meeting when the whole office gathered into the large meeting area to run through a plethora of items on the agenda that could easily have been tackled in an email (you know the score, I'm sure).

I was squeezed around the table, in between two of my colleagues, and the room was particularly hot and stuffy. It was silent, apart from the low murmur of the air conditioning unit (which clearly wasn't working) and the host of the meeting, who spoke very… very quietly.

Suddenly, my stomach decided it had had enough. A loud burping/farting sound emerged from the depths of my bowels and I almost shot out of my seat in mortification. There were beads of sweat on my forehead from embarrassment and panic, the fear that I would be shunned by my colleagues and the strain of being on high alert in case I needed to dash out and run to the toilet. It was awful. After about ten minutes, I grabbed my paperwork and fled the meeting room. I then plonked myself on the toilet and cried.

The worst thing was that I didn't even NEED the toilet. I was constipated. I hadn't been for days. So my body didn't even reward me with a poo after all that trauma. I still felt bloated, ginormous and totally miserable.

I later discovered that this gassy, empty, farty and constipated Scarlett creation was a direct result of consuming dairy (see other chapters for further details). The effect it has on me is what I like to fondly refer to as 'empty poos'. So you get all the signs, the urges and the gas. But no end result. Nothing to show for it. If you know what I mean.

I can literally be sitting on the toilet for three hours popping away and nothing will come out and I will have no relief from the cramping, gas and bloatedness. It's marvellous. Especially when it decides to creep up on me during a busy meeting.

After that particular episode, I began fearing that it would happen again, and so I avoided situations I couldn't easily escape from.

It got to the point that it was so bad, I was having to either work from home or call in sick, or a mixture of the two. I felt so guilty. I was letting people down. I felt that I would be seen as unreliable and I couldn't properly do the job I LOVED doing. And worst of all, there was nothing I could do about it. I felt like my body was dictating and driving my every move, without my consent.

Thankfully, my line manager was very understanding and really genuinely cared about my wellbeing. We came up with a flexible working arrangement that meant, I could work from home and tune into meetings via Skype if I was going through a particularly bad flare up. (That way, if I needed to dash to the loo, I could just close the laptop and blame connection problems, though thankfully I never needed to do this).

She enabled me to come in just for mornings or afternoons and work the rest of the day from home. She also left the door open for me whenever we had meetings. I was still in the meeting room, but the door wasn't closed and oddly, this was SO incredibly helpful as it put my mind at ease. I felt the 'open door' policy meant I could dash to the loo and there was no faffing around with the door handle and drawing attention to myself. I could dash out unnoticed.

Often help is just a question away, and in all aspects of my life, I have come to realise that you just have to ASK for the things you need. More often than not, people are more than happy to accommodate. I used to believe that if you alluded to something, or subtly hinted, the other person would telepathically understand what it is you were asking for. But usually, my questions, queries and concerns were lost in translation. The only way you're really able to get what you need is to ask for it explicitly. Don't be shy!

I think the most daunting thing I faced after initially finding out about IBS was that I had to suffer with it alone. For the first 6-7 years, I didn't tell a soul about my IBS, apart from my mum. I isolated myself out of fear I would be 'found out' and that people would think I was disgusting and weird. Navigating school life is difficult enough in itself, let alone doing it with a chronic bowel condition too.

But once I started opening up about what I was going through, I soon realised that there were not only others who were suffering from the same thing, but also help and support available.

After a year of working and figuring out the traditional 9-5 life wasn't what I expected it to be, I decided to go full steam ahead with university. Luckily, because I had deferred and already had my place on my course, I could apply for a place at halls before anyone else. So I put my name down on the list for a room with a private bathroom.

Before I knew it, I was packing up my things and travelling 120 miles away to Bournemouth, where I was to begin the next chapter of my life.

I will never forget my parents helping me to unpack and then, suddenly, I was in this brand new room, all by myself, and I realised I knew no-one. Not a soul.

I suppose the stress of being miles away from home, without my immediate support system in place was a little overwhelming and so, of course, my IBS symptoms decided to come along for the ride too.

Then, after just one week, I had another blow to the system – my relationship of four years ended.

This whole saga was a huge upset to me and culminated in the worst flare-up I've ever had. We'll talk about love and the perils of romance and dating when you have IBS in another section, but this experience meant that I really struggled with my symptoms in a strange and unfamiliar place. As a result, this was even more of a challenge than anything I'd experienced previously.

The lecture theatres at university were even more intimidating than the classrooms I was used to at school. They were vast, intimidating, cold and quiet. Plus the door was just adjacent to the stage where the professor stood, so you couldn't leave without the entire theatre (of up to 400 people) turning to look at you and wondering why you were leaving early.

I absolutely dreaded lectures and really struggled to take on board what was being said when all I could think about was my stomach. Or worse still, keeling over in pain.

Again, thankfully, I felt confident enough to ask for help and so I visited the Learning Support Advice service (located in the library) for assistance. They arranged a separate exam room for me, as well as pointing me in the direction of the 'Student Disability Allowance' (SDA)*.

*This may have all changed since I graduated (and, bear in mind, this is just applicable for the UK – so it may be worth researching similar programs in your college/university).

After an initial assessment, the SDA granted me with a new laptop so that I could do all the work I needed to do from my student bedroom if I was too poorly to go in. My old laptop was on its last legs and certainly not equipped with the kind of processing ability that my journalism and multi-media course required (where work was completed on Apple Mac computers). They also spoke to the library about extending the time I was allowed to take books out.

In addition to the above, they also funded me to have a note-taker who was able to attend lectures on my behalf if I was too unwell to attend a lesson or lecture. This was a huge reassurance as I felt an overwhelming amount of guilt whenever I missed a session, and this gave me the opportunity to stay on top of my work and not worry about whether I was bound to the bathroom that day or not.

Now running my own business, I am sympathetic to each person's individual requirements when having meetings. I often suggest Skype conferences where the pressure is taken off and I'm in the comfort of my own environment, or if the meeting has to be face-to-face, I choose a busy coffee shop. There have been occasions where I've still had to enter quiet formal meeting rooms, but I have certain coping mechanisms to deal with this situation that I have learned through CBT. Often, it's good to try 'exposing' yourself to the fear, as well as making arrangements for more comfortable environments. Striking a balance between the two can be a really productive way of accommodating your symptoms, without letting them control your working life.

In the end, although I found no 'miracle' solution, I tried to not feel as guilty when I had to work from home or miss a meeting. I would make up for it in other ways, such as working harder to fulfil a brief or putting in the hours elsewhere. In meetings that I couldn't miss or days when I HAD to be in, I'd take little snacks and a big bottle of water in with me. This usually helped to keep things as under control as possible. I do think having other people know about the condition would have helped, but in hindsight, I wasn't confident enough at that point to talk about it.

Despite this, however, I have never ever thought to myself, 'Ah, you know what, I'll just give up with this lark.' By lark, I mean work. It is tough. It's tough enough being successful in a job full stop, let alone when you have another factor to add to the equation. You might find yourself choosing your career path based solely on your IBS. But please don't let that be the case. Your IBS shouldn't be allowed to define you. When you have a hold on it (and it WILL happen), you don't want to regret not fulfilling the path your destined for. But then again, it's not worth being dreadfully unhappy in a career where you are suffering too. It's a very difficult balance. But I'm determined to be successful in my chosen career – journalism, with or without the extra hurdle of IBS. You WILL find ways around things. It's just a matter of when. My mum has always been the strongest advocate for me in terms of not letting my IBS rule my life. And although it does at times, it won't rule where I want my career to take me. And it won't rule my success. I'm determined about that. I just hope I'm right.

I often worry when I tell people I have IBS, they will think less of me. Think that I'm unreliable. Be wary of hiring me. It's not necessarily something you'd mention in a job interview anyway. But at the end of the day, I think it is natural to have bouts of the IBS being bad. Focus on the good. Focus on making sure that you are the best you can possibly be. When you're next at work, look around the room and wonder how many others might be suffering in silence too. Or glance around and wonder whether they would deal with IBS symptoms as gracefully and as well as you are. You're still here. You're still working. So you should be proud of yourself. And even if your IBS did get to the point where you had to quit work, as many of you were telling me about on Twitter – don't feel guilty. Pick yourself up, you'll soon be back on track. Focus instead on being the best that you can be. Whatever that is.

COULD YOU REQUEST A MORE FLEXIBLE WORKING PATTERN?

Perhaps your symptoms are worse in the mornings and better in the early afternoon. It's always worth talking to your boss or line manager and trying to come to an arrangement that fits you and accommodates your needs. At the end of the day, if your boss wants (and needs) to get the best from you, they should be able to come to a logical compromise. Perhaps this is in the form of working from home for a few days a week, or even something as simple as having your desk moved nearer to the bathroom. Don't be afraid of asking for help, it is out there – you just have to be bold and request it.

DON'T SEE YOUR IBS AS A 'FLAW', SEE IT AS A MOTIVATION

We all have ebbs and flows of motivation throughout our lives. We might find that when we have goals to work towards, our work ethic and productivity is higher. For me personally, my IBS is a constant motivation to push forward and achieve what I wish to strive for. Try to retrain your mind to see your IBS as a motivator, and not as a flaw or a problem.

REMEMBER TO STAY HYDRATED AND MOVE YOUR BODY

I used to find that being hunched over an office desk all day was enough to kick-start awful stomach cramps by lunchtime, which would then continue until I left at 5pm. Remember to put your body first and exercise self-care, even when you're in the office. It really helped me to have a drawer at my desk where I had a peppermint tea stash, a bottle of water and some healthy snacks. I'd make sure to stretch my legs every half an hour and fill up my water bottle.

DON'T TRY TO BE PERFECT

I actually won an award aged 14 for being the 'class perfectionist', with each accolade of the award listed on the certificate: the neatest textbook, the neatest handwriting etc. I never wanted to disappoint my teachers and I so desperately wanted to be liked and told that I was doing well. So I tried to be perfect at everything and always felt deeply ashamed when I'd fail, fall short or wasn't picked for something. Sidenote: to provide some context for the latter, I was never picked for anything, despite committing to the cause and bringing in a full-sized BROOM to school with me for an *Annie* production audition. I was cast as a 'homeless person' rather than the star part that I had gone for originally.

I took any deemed 'failure' as a direct insult to myself. This is totally silly I know, but when you're young and riddled with anxiety, small critiques or comments seemed like the end of the world. So my advice is not to attempt perfection, or even anywhere close to it. The mistakes you make and the lessons you learn along the way are far more valuable than any seemingly successful attempt at being perfect. When you have IBS you sometimes feel like you have to work EXTRA hard to make up for the things you don't have control over, which can unintentionally worsen your symptoms. But just do your best and know when to switch off from work/studying/school. Everyone needs balance!

My parents have been immensely helpful and understanding with my IBS battles, especially during the initial years when I had no idea why these hideous symptoms were plaguing my body.

I know it was very difficult for my mum at times to see me so upset, wishing for a 'normal body' and crying out in pain, because there was nothing she could do to immediately relieve what I was going through.

My mum, in particular, spent years researching solutions. We spent many evenings together, both in tears, because of how much I was struggling. She took me to hypnotherapy, spent hours of an evening making special gluten-free dishes for me to take into school the following day and spent countless hours consoling me and reassuring me that I would be okay.

She still remains my biggest cheerleader and an incredible support system. I know that I'm very lucky to have such a wonderful, kind and caring mum who has never disregarded my symptoms or told me they were 'all in my head'. It can be difficult for other people around you to really understand what you are going through when the symptoms are totally invisible, so it takes a really loving, heartfelt approach to make the sufferer feel like they are being listened to.

When putting this book together, I had a very frank, honest and open chat with her about how she coped with my initial IBS diagnosis. Whether you are considering how to approach telling your parents or guardian about your symptoms - or whether you are a parent yourself who is faced with a child who suffers from IBS - I thought it would be helpful to pop it below, in its raw form.

When do you remember me first complaining of tummy troubles?

Scarlett is an intelligent, creative, organised, quite serious girl with a kind nature; however, she has always been a bit of a worrier and sensitive too. She was happy at Primary School and did well. She really looked forward to starting Senior School. Indeed, I remember her first day – she bounced out of bed at 5.30am, got dressed and had her new school uniform, complete with backpack on by 6.30am, all ready to leave! She made a nice group of friends and I don't remember any real issues or worries at school until she reached 14.

It began when she came home one day and told me that she was getting the feeling of "bubbling and gurgling" in her tummy during the school day and a weird uncomfortable feeling. She was conscious of her tummy making really loud noises during class, which she was really concerned everyone would hear. At first, I reassured her that it was the normal function of the stomach and they were just tummy rumbles – everyone's stomach makes noises when they are hungry but she was quite upset about it and said it was really embarrassing. I kept reiterating to her that it was normal and nothing at all to worry about.

However, over the next week or two, she became more and more anxious about it and every day would come home from school quite upset. She had some exams coming up so I put it down to her starting to worry about the exams. Scarlett has always worked very hard at school so I never had to remind her to do her homework or study for exams. I think the anxiousness started to really become a problem at this point. She would be in tears and needed a lot of reassurance.

I would sit her down and give her a cuddle, sympathise, listen to her worries and concerns and try to keep her calm. I suggested that maybe we should look at what she was eating at school. We sat together and researched her symptoms on the internet and found articles about there being a link with anxiety and gurgling, uncomfortable stomach pains. I had suffered from a couple of episodes in the past and so I suggested trying peppermint tea, which helped a bit.

After school, we would talk about everything she had eaten that day and, at this point, I think we talked about how certain foods might be upsetting her tummy and potentially trying to cut out certain foods.

The exams were still looming and Scarlett would say to me, "Mum I know how important these exams are – I feel so much pressure about them!" I truly believe this is where it all started – school exams pressure, coupled with the fact that she has an anxious nature, which is exacerbated by outside stresses. As a young, intelligent, sensitive teenage girl who was a real worrier, it was difficult to reassure her.

The emotional upset was difficult to deal with. It was happening most days and I felt awful, that I was failing her as a mum as I just couldn't make her feel better. I was really upset and worried – why was this happening to her, was it serious? – but tried not to show Scarlett because I didn't want to add to her worries by letting her think I was scared. All I could do was to be sympathetic and loving to her, and to talk it through with her and let her cry. I just reassured her over and over again that it was just anxiousness and she should try not to worry, but I started to feel really frustrated and helpless.

She then started to get more pain and diarrhoea so I took her to see the GP.

Do you remember the first doctor's visit to do with IBS – what prompted it?

I think the GP told us that gut symptoms can be linked to anxiety and can speed up the metabolism, hence the rumbles and noises could be associated with hunger. So I would give you cereal bars to take to school to eat during breaks to stave off hunger and avoid getting trapped wind, so it wouldn't get worse. At that point, I think the GP did some blood tests to see if you were coeliac, which came back as normal, and prescribed Buscopan or Mebeverine.

However, over the course of a few months, I could feel it was becoming more of an issue and was starting to cause her more anxiety. She would ring me over the weekend when she stayed at her Dad's house, crying and sobbing about it. I was in tears too as I just wanted to make it all go away. She begged me to speak to the school because she became convinced that the whole class could hear her stomach noises. As the exams were coming up, she just couldn't face sitting in a completely silent classroom as she wouldn't be able to concentrate on her exams because of the overriding fear of the noises – she was petrified everyone would hear and start to make fun of her. It was really hard to convince her – no matter how hard we all tried – that no-one was bothered and it wasn't unusual. She kept saying, no-one else has this – nobody understands how I feel. It sounds so trivial but to her, it was her whole world and she couldn't shake it off. I would spend ages sitting with her, hugging, with us both in tears wondering what the problem was. We pondered again whether to cut out food groups and sat at the computer researching what caused weird tummy noises and an uncomfortable, painful tummy.

I contacted her teacher, who was very understanding. Her main concern was that other pupils would be able to hear her stomach noises, so she was really worried and asked me to ask if you could sit her exams in a separate room. Scarlett's teacher agreed. We had to provide a doctor's letter as evidence. I felt hugely relieved that they had agreed to take her concerns seriously and she seemed happier that she would be able to sit in a separate room.

How was it for you to see me struggling with the symptoms, but being somewhat powerless to help?

It was really hard because the medication hadn't helped, in fact, it made it worse because this is when the pain started.

We went back to the GP once or twice again and he referred you to a Paediatric Consultant. We saw a doctor who examined you and felt your tummy. She diagnosed severe constipation and impaction (the medication prescribed to relieve the diarrhoea symptoms had, in fact, made you constipated, so you were then in pain because you were constipated). She prescribed stuff to make you go to the loo! Unfortunately, because you had previously had diarrhoea, you were reluctant to take this. So it took a while to sort out and we needed to understand the process of it all. It was a very frustrating and confusing time. At times, we would argue because I was trying to support you but you wouldn't always stick to the regime, or wouldn't take the medication and so we couldn't really ever see much improvement. I felt utterly helpless, frustrated to see my beautiful daughter so distraught and that I couldn't fix it.

I think, at this point, you decided that it might be linked to diet and I suggested cutting out gluten, wheat and/or dairy. However, you only ever stuck to it for a week or so which was frustrating. But equally, as a mum of a young girl still growing, I wasn't entirely comfortable either with you restricting certain food groups due to the potential risk of a lack of certain dietary foods/nutrients, etc. so we were always trying to find ways to manage the problem.

I'm pretty certain things always got better during the holidays (the symptoms were at their worse at university and you never suffered as badly at home).

You didn't ever once convince me that my IBS symptoms weren't real or that it was all in my head. How important is it for a parent to validate their child's IBS and try to understand it?

During your school years, I didn't believe it was necessarily a serious illness as such, and it seemed mostly attributable to exam times and worrying what other kids would think if they heard your tummy noises but it was a big issue for you so, of course, I wanted to reassure you and listen to your worries and concerns and try to allay your fears but I hoped you would grow out of it.

However, when you were at university it got worse. You would ring me in floods of tears, saying you couldn't face sitting in the lecture halls because it was so embarrassing to have to keep rushing out to go to the toilet, and you were in a lot of pain.

Fortunately, you were able to get notes taken and it's testament to your hard work that you gained a First Class Degree despite all this. However, I then really began to worry when the diarrhoea got so much worse and that you were in crippling pain. All I could do at that time was to speak to you over the phone, try to calm you down and talk you through it. I kept reassuring you and suggested ways to help you cope with it but it was awful for you and a huge worry for me as you were away from home and suffering so terribly. Actually, this was the WORST time.

I just wanted to drive to your university, put you in my car and wrap you up and take you home, but it is such an important thing and I was just trying to keep you strong by talking you through it and showing as much support as I could, albeit remotely. I will never forget those terrible phone calls where you were literally sobbing on the phone and I was in bits because I just couldn't do anything to help you. However, you struggled on, as I knew you would, and you had to get through the days when it wasn't so bad; and when it was, you stayed in bed with a hot water bottle and worked on your laptop. You never gave up though and I am so incredibly proud that you managed to keep going. I think you had to talk me out of driving down there in the middle of the night to console you. I was at the end of my tether at that point, it was hideous – you were suffering so much. However, you are tougher than you think and said, 'Mum I will carry on.' There was no doubt in my mind that you wouldn't succeed but it certainly wasn't easy.

It is crucial for parents to listen and take their child's concerns seriously, sympathise, and try and find ways to help control the symptoms and explore every avenue possible.

The turning point was when Scarlett had the endoscopy privately – despite it being a horrible, invasive procedure. Once we got the results, which were thankfully all normal, and the gastroenterologist was reassuring. I felt that a weight had been lifted. At that point, Scarlett had already started cutting out certain foods and things were already getting a little better.

Is there anything during that time period (from when I was first diagnosed until I was about 15-16) that you would have done differently?

Not really, I don't think we could have done anything else – we literally tried everything we could! I was at work one day, researching once again, and found a Harley Street Hypnotherapist who specialised in IBS, so I took you there when you were about 15 or 16. He recorded a CD for you to listen to at night and before exams. However, each time we tried something new it would help for a bit, as I think we both felt it was a positive move to try different methods to help cope – however, it didn't cure the IBS. It is a case of finding ways to manage symptoms so that when the episodes come, sufferers can put their own methods in place to cope with those times.

Do you think the emotional aspect of IBS isn't as widely discussed as it should be?

No, it isn't, especially for younger children or teenagers. It is vitally important they can relate to others, so reading or hearing about it might stop the cycle of the symptoms linked to anxiety. But it's also important not to overload them with too much information.

What advice would you give to other mums who have children suffering from IBS?

Be there to reassure them, listen to their worries and concerns, be sympathetic but give practical solutions, offer to research foods and plan meals. Just be their support system.

- O   TRY TO SUGGEST COPING MECHANISMS.
- O   TRY TO IDENTIFY IF CERTAIN FOODS TRIGGER SYMPTOMS.
- O   PERHAPS TRY A PROBIOTIC.

I'll never forget the hideous words uttered to me by a guy I was dating several years ago. We hadn't been seeing one another for long and I was eager to make a good impression.

"I'll cook you dinner at my house."

CHAPTER 7

Dating & Intimacy

(Originally published on Healthline)

Most women, I assume, would find this terribly romantic. A man, a home-cooked dinner, a cosy evening in.

But for me, this invitation was my biggest nightmare.

I also had another factor to add to the evening, though albeit a less romantic one.

IBS.

Sitting at his dining table, with no background chatter to mask the noises my stomach would be making as it bubbled away nervously.

No distractions to comfort the fact that I might need to dash to the toilet several times an hour.

No immediate escape should I enter into a horribly uncontrollable flare-up where my digestive symptoms might ruin the night altogether.

Nope, unfortunately for me, this terribly romantic cliché was my idea of dating hell.

Irritable Bowel Syndrome and dating, as a whole, don't really mix. Do they?

There's nothing that makes you feel sexier than worrying about your bowels.

Can you detect the sarcasm?

If you're a sufferer too, then you probably have also experienced the nightmare that can proceed when IBS and an attempt to navigate the dating scene are woven together. It can be rather tricky, but it's not impossible.

I'm now in a long-term relationship with a wonderfully loving man who has changed my outlook on the condition and how I view it with regards to my romantic life.

It really doesn't need to interfere, so here's what you need to remember when you're dating and managing your digestive symptoms.

TAKE CONTROL

When it comes to IBS, we all know that, unfortunately, we often have very little control over the symptoms themselves. We can minimise a flare-up by steering clear of our triggers, managing stress and exercising regularly, but of course, the unpredictability of the condition means that you can never be totally sure. So, when it comes to dating, take control of the one thing you can have the ultimate decision over – where, when and how. Suggest restaurants that you know you can eat in and pick a noisy place, so you don't have to worry about tummy grumbles or wind, and make sure that you're as prepared as you can be, so you'll know where the toilets are should the worst occur. This often helps to put our mind at rest while the dating is very new and extra scary, and means you won't feel awkward in your surroundings.

BE HONEST EARLY ON

Admittedly, announcing: "I have IBS which means I might spend long amounts of time on this date in the toilet," isn't exactly a winning opening line. But when the moment is right, whether it's the first date or the second, I would be honest about your digestive troubles rather than keeping it to yourself until further down the line. It's always easier to broach the subject early on. It's not only a good tester of character to see how they react, but it also means you're not keeping your symptoms a secret – which can often be just as stressful as managing them. Being open, honest and upfront can help you to feel much more relaxed on subsequent dates – and considering it affects 10 to 20% of the Western world, you might even find that your date suffers too. My current boyfriend put me at instant ease on our third date when he (unfortunately or fortunately, you can be the judge) ate something a bit dodgy and explained rather openly about his own digestive troubles. It helped to reassure me that he wasn't judging me for my bowel issues and that we all have stuff going on internally that we don't always share initially!

ACCEPT THAT NOT EVERYONE WILL UNDERSTAND

Just like no two dates are exactly the same, no two people will react in exactly the same way to your IBS struggles. Some people are terribly sympathetic, some engage you in their own life story, some trivialise your symptoms and others are downright confused as to what on earth IBS is. I remember a date once where I explained about my 'sensitive stomach' only to receive a rather unkind response which involved eye rolling and an announcement that, "Oh, so you're one of those hypochondriacs then". It's safe to say, there wasn't a second date. But while it was a little upsetting initially, it made me realise that not everyone understands and often his or her initial reaction will be an insightful first impression of someone's character.

DON'T FEEL EMBARRASSED

Remember that everyone has their strengths and everyone has their weaknesses. It doesn't make you weaker to have IBS, but everyone has aspects of their character and body that they love – and others that they aren't so keen on. But they all add up to make you what you are, so own it! You shouldn't feel embarrassed about your IBS, it's just another part of you, and the right person will understand! It's easy to focus on the negatives and believe that IBS is a burden in some way (and yes, admittedly it's not great) but have confidence in your own wonderfulness. Your body might be high maintenance but it's no less fantastic or desirable!

BE KIND TO YOURSELF

The symptoms of IBS, gas, bloating, diarrhoea, constipation are nuisances that everyone has suffered from at some time or another, if not regularly. So while they might not have to deal with them at the same intensity that you do, they will understand that these symptoms are not a reflection on you as a person. The fact that everyone has had experience with the unpleasantness of the symptoms means that they will not be judging you as harshly as you think. So if you do end up spending more time in the bathroom than you want to, most (good) people will be sympathetic to your quandary. Make sure you apply the same kindness to yourself.

ASK FOR HELP

I remember one absolutely awful dating experience with my first boyfriend, when we set off for our first holiday at his family's holiday home in Europe. I had no idea what the bathroom situation would be like; whether we'd have our own ensuite or be sharing with the rest of his siblings and parents. But nothing had prepared me for the situation that awaited. Not only did the toilet door have a transparent pane of glass running the length of it (with just a flimsy curtain to protect your modesty) but there was also a hole in the wall that led through to the hallway, where everyone congregated before and after meals.

I spent the entire week trying to sneak off to a public toilet and keep my troubles a secret. Really, I should have asked for help or confided in someone on the trip because having to worry about where I was going to be able to go to the toilet in private made my symptoms even worse. Plus, if I'd asked for help, someone might have been able to give me an alternative option to make me feel more comfortable. Following the trip, I vowed never to keep things to myself again!

KNOW WHEN TO LAUGH

Obviously, for the most part, IBS isn't a laughing matter. It's hardly hilarious when you're cramped over the toilet for the fourth time that morning, wondering if you'll ever be able to leave the house because you're having a flare-up. Nor is it side-splittingly funny when you're doubled over in pain because you have trapped wind or severe bloating. However, in order to let your personality shine through behind the serious protective blanket that IBS can form, you do need to know when to laugh sometimes. Laughing and poking a bit of fun at your own IBS can really help you to overcome the internal embarrassment it can often create. If your stomach makes a funny sound, lighten your mood a little rather than stressing out about it by saying, "I've got a lion in my tummy today" or "my stomach says pass the salt please". Sometimes, laughter is the best medicine!

CHOOSE YOUR OUTFIT WISELY

Obviously, when you're venturing off to a first date, you want to dress to impress. But as someone with digestive struggles knows all too well, you often dress for your IBS too. Pick something that you're going to be comfortable wearing and feel good in. I would definitely recommend not wearing tight jeans as there is a chance the food in a restaurant may cause a reaction, and I've been in the unfortunate situation so many times where I've practically had to peel my jeans away from my stomach to relieve the agonising pain. Tight clothes and IBS don't always mix. But I'd always recommend having a 'go-to' outfit for dating that you know you're going to feel sexy and comfortable in. For me, it's a little black dress in a size bigger than I normally take. I accentuate my waist using a thin belt, but if I start feeling my stomach going, I can quite easily whip the belt off and enjoy the floaty, light material that covers any bloating and isn't tight around my tummy.

Managing your IBS struggles on the side can be a very good (albeit unintentional) date filter, as you wade through the good and the bad dates, based on how they react to your explanation of your symptoms.

Not everyone will understand, but the right person will!

And that's the oddly great thing about IBS – it's an in-built filter for both friends and romantic relationships, as you quickly figure out who is worth your time and who most definitely isn't.

If someone isn't able to, at the very least, try and empathise with your plight, then it's a red flag they might not be right for you.

My current boyfriend actually broached the subject with me on our third date after reading ALL about my IBS (including some rather fabulous TMI details about how many bowel movements I had per day) on my blog. So I didn't ever actually have to bring the subject up with him or try and awkwardly explain it.

He was incredible about it, put me at complete ease, and told me I could chat to him about it at any time and he'd be there to listen.

To this day, he has been the most supportive person I could ever wish for and without getting overly gushing, I couldn't wish for a better human to share my life with.

Almost instantly, he proved his kind, loving and caring qualities by acting in this way and I can totally relax around him.

He understands my food intolerances and always asks the waiters before going into a restaurant on my behalf, so I don't have to make it a big deal. He will know instantly if I'm suffering from pain or trapped wind and he'll bring me up a peppermint tea or a hot water bottle, or cancel a social engagement without even having to ask.

So, rest assured, there are people out there who will understand and treat you with the kindness (and IBS empathy) you need and deserve.

But there are also people who won't and, luckily, IBS is a great buffer that will quickly notify if someone might be right or wrong for you.

In the case of someone being COMPLETELY wrong for you, I present to you my infamous 'tomato-gate' story. It's not so much about IBS symptoms, but more about my food intolerances. (That if I ate said food, my IBS symptoms would rear their ugly heads, so it's all the same thing, I suppose.)

I had informed my date prior to meeting him of my various intolerances and he seemed relatively understanding, suggesting a couple of places that I assumed he'd eaten in before and knew would be quite flexible for dairy-free me.

I arrived at the restaurant in question, greeted the guy and had a quick look at the menu outside (it was one of those places that was 'too exclusive' to put a menu up online so I couldn't pre-plan my meal beforehand). Immediately, it was apparent that there was nothing on the menu I could eat.

It's awkward enough on a first date, without not being able to eat, so I politely asked whether we might be able to try a different restaurant as I wasn't going to be able to eat anything. Much to my surprise, he put his foot down and insisted that we eat at THIS particular restaurant.

So we ventured inside and were seated at a table. As I had imagined, they were not very accommodating or flexible with their menu. I sat at the table and ordered a side plate of tomatoes. TOMATOES. Because that was ALL I could have.

They were vine tomatoes, not particularly juicy and one was slightly mushy and looked like it had seen better days. If you were wondering.

But my gracious date wasn't put off by my measly plate of tomatoes and took full advantage of the menu by ordering THREE COURSES. Oh yes. Starter, main AND dessert.

The best part came when we split the bill and he suggested 'we go halves'.

I'm far too polite and – I'm ashamed to say – I actually paid half and left as quickly as I could.

But it certainly taught me a lesson about calling up the restaurant beforehand and checking out the menu and their flexibility.

And also choosing my dates more wisely.

I also have a rather delightful alien-wind-grumble-stomach-noise story which happened when I was 15. I was round a friend's house, on the sofa watching a film and about to go in for the kiss with the boy sitting next to me when suddenly, from the inner depths of my bowels came an almighty whale noise. Yes, a WHALE noise.

If we'd have been watching *Free Willy* I might have got away with it. But unfortunately we were punishing ourselves with a hideous horror film (I've blanked out which one it was) and my stomach decided to say hello during a particularly tense silent moment. It certainly knows when to make an appearance, eh?

The moral of the story is, don't rule out finding someone who understands. Because there is someone out there who does understand and you will find them.

Dating is difficult with the added pressure of IBS symptoms flaring up, but as I said, it's a great filter of who is lovely and who isn't, and being honest early on is key. The best relationships flourish when both parties feel comfortable, safe and cared for. So keep this in mind.

Communication is key to defeating any issues that may arise within a relationship.

Shame and secrecy are intimacy killers, both emotionally and sexually. Being frank and unembarrassed about your stomach issues in the context of an intimate relationship is the key to success.

If you are struggling to broach the subject with a potential suitor, writing down what you want to say can really help to get the message across, without any emotions getting in the way or missing anything out. You could write your other half a letter explaining exactly how you feel, then let them read it, or you could read it out loud to them.

Some of you have reached out to let me know that you've even grabbed your laptop, popped on my YouTube Video (the video is titled 'We need to talk about this - IBS'), plonked it in front of your friend/family member/partner and let them watch it from start to finish. This can act as a means of allowing them to understand IBS and other related digestive symptoms from a voice that isn't yours, as well as highlighting that there are others experiencing the same inner turmoil as you.

And regardless of this, any dating disasters are always great stories to tell! So there's always that!

Because I want this book to be a helpful guide for all parties involved in your IBS journey, I thought I would put together a section where my boyfriend can answer some questions regarding what it's like to be a partner of a sufferer.

As I mentioned before, I've been very lucky with how kind and supportive my partner is because I know it's not always the case and I empathise with how tricky it is to broach the subject with your other half, especially in the early days.

David has been my rock whenever I've been having a flare-up, fetching my mugs of peppermint tea, bringing me hot water bottles in bed and giving me his famous 'tummy rubs' (usually just an excuse to get him to stroke me – anyone else LOVE being stroked, massaged or having your hair played with – just me then?).

He even seems to have developed a psychic ability to know exactly WHEN I am suffering from a flare-up or having a panic attack because he immediately, and discreetly, reaches over to hold my hand and reminds me to breathe slowly and deeply.

When did you first discover that I had IBS and how did it make you feel?

I discovered that you had IBS about three weeks or so before I actually met you. I remember reading your very honest and open blog posts that detailed your symptoms and struggles with IBS. It didn't change my opinion whatsoever and had no effect on how much I liked you. However, I did know that I wanted to broach the subject with you early on, to hopefully put you at ease. I wanted to make sure you could have a lovely time on our first few dates without worrying about addressing it and potentially triggering a flare-up as a result. I knew from your blog posts that you preferred being open about it but found it difficult to bring it up initially, so I took the pressure off by bringing it up myself. We broke the ice in the initial stages and I think that helped you relax. I also ate cauliflower on our second date, one of my 'trigger foods', and so my stomach started chatting away to yours during a quiet moment together and we both laughed. I think my stomach was trying to chat yours up!

What was your understanding of IBS?

To be honest, my knowledge of IBS was relatively little in comparison to now. Until you've been close to someone who is suffering from severe symptoms of IBS it is difficult to totally appreciate and understand the impact it can have on an individual. I am still very much learning but am definitely more aware of the triggers for it and how different forms of management can be effective.

Does my IBS affect our life together – if so, how? Are you aware of anything you actively do to make it easier for me to live with IBS?

I'm very careful about food selection and I always check food labels, ingredients and restaurant allergen menus.

When initially introducing you to my family and friends, I discussed your food intolerances before you met with them so that they were aware ahead of time and could plan any food related arrangements accordingly. I think everyone was really accommodating and I remember one Christmas my family practically purchased the entire 'Free From' section from the local supermarket because they weren't sure what you could and couldn't eat. The term IBS wasn't mentioned until much further down the line when you were more comfortable talking about it openly with them.

I try my best to make every experience as stress-free and 'normal' for you, because I would hate for you to ever feel awkward and as a result, potentially trigger your symptoms by worrying about a certain situation. There have been occasions when you've felt too poorly to attend a social event and so I ring ahead and tell them we won't be making it. It's sometimes easier to make a decision like that myself because struggling through it can only make you feel worse

- sometimes it's better to rest at home. I also like to think I am 'chief-hot-water-bottle-maker' of the house, a simple role that I know can really ease painful stomach cramps and provide a little bit of relief for you.

Me being calm and reassuring definitely helps as it's not nice to see anyone in pain or uncomfortable, let alone my girl-friend – the person who I love. Whenever you get a bout of symptoms, I often think I'd love to trade places with you so that you would not be in pain.

Did my IBS ever 'put you off' me?

Not at all. You are such a wonderful person and I love you for every individual thing that makes up your being. Everyone has their own individual health issues and there is no need to ever be embarrassed of them. You shouldn't be judged on one thing that affects you in your daily life. I know you have to juggle so many aspects of life - on top of IBS. I'm so proud that you manage to balance everything so well and that only makes me admire you even more!

Do you ever find my IBS gross?

No, I think it's just another part of you which is unique. At the end of the day, going to the toilet is a normal daily occurrence for everyone on this planet. Taboo often means that society is embarrassed by talking about topics. However, really we should embrace it as more people suffer from the symptoms than maybe let on. So being open and honest is probably the best way of crushing the taboo subject and making IBS a well-researched, backed and public topic. It's natural and yet just slightly different. We should not think a normal yet slightly different bodily function is gross because if that was the case then no-one in society would feel comfortable. Just be open-minded and honest while feeling empathy and sympathy for your fellow human being as that can help the situation hugely, especially because of the anxiety surrounding the subject.

Has the fact that I've been so open with you regarding my IBS made you more open with me about your own personal issues?

Being open and honest in a relationship is key, so yes, it has made me feel more relaxed in sharing any problems I have with you and perhaps it has brought us closer as a couple. Being in a relationship, you are there for one another and it's wonderful to have a support system within a best friend! There shouldn't be anything that you feel you have to hide or shy away from.

Do you have any advice for other people whose partners are also IBS sufferers?

Comfort, support and empathy. Understanding your partner is key and if you don't understand, then ask them how they feel and what you could do to help and make their experience a better one the next time it happens, or is about to happen. That could then change their opinion on the matter and they will feel the love and support, which I find is key to the situation.

My job involves a lot of travel, which is incredibly fun but, of course, IBS can make things a teeny bit more complex.

CHAPTER 8

Travel

This chapter features material originally published on Healthline.

n the past year, I've travelled to St Lucia, Venice, Cyprus, Los Angeles, Las Vegas, Mexico, Singapore and Paris.

Not only do I have to prepare for every digestive eventuality within the confines of my suitcase but I also have to make sure I'm fit and ready to work, as so much of my job involves taking photos and wearing lots of fancy clothes, which isn't always ideal when you're feeling pretty bloated.

Time differences, jet lag and air pressure can play havoc with your usual symptoms, so I always like to be as equipped as possible should my IBS kick up a fuss.

As anyone with IBS will know, lack of control is a huge factor in stressing out our symptoms. We never know when a flare-up will occur – and that's scary.

So I find that planning the things I CAN actually control as much as possible helps to relax me and really puts my mind at ease.

That's not to say I haven't been caught out on occasions. I remember one fateful time that occurred during a long haul trip to Thailand that I took with my boyfriend David.

We'd just checked into a beautiful luxurious hotel in Khanom, a remote part of Thailand that offers serene coast-line, unspoiled views and a tranquil, undiscovered experience unlike no other. Sorry, I'm starting to sound like a travel brochure here - but I'm sure you get the idea. We were in a gorgeous place, and typically, my IBS decided to say hello.

Our luxurious villa for the four days we were there was absolutely stunning; we had our own pool which led directly onto the beachfront with panoramic views of the ocean. We had a huge four-poster bed and an incredible marble open plan bathroom.

As an added 'extra', the bathroom had shutters which opened out into the bedroom, so you could enjoy the stunning view, detailed above, from the comfort of your… toilet.

I definitely appreciated the sentiment initially, but when I felt explosive diarrhoea ready to erupt from inside the confines of my stomach at 2am, I suddenly wished that we had a far more 'traditional' hotel room.

I remember waking up in the middle of the night and feeling an almighty sense of dread in my stomach, as I wasn't quite at the level of 'comfort' in my relationship yet where I could confidently sit on the toilet and unleash whatever was inside me with my new boyfriend peacefully sleeping right in front of the open shutters.

In fact, I'm not sure I'll ever be at quite THAT level of comfort.

So I did what any refined IBS sufferer would do at 2am in a remote Thai resort. I crept out of the villa, in search of a toilet with a little more… privacy.

And, unfortunately, I almost pooped en route as I stumbled upon a giant lizard (I believe they are actually called Monitor Lizards, they can grow up to 6ft long and are seemingly unfazed by half-asleep women running across their path clenching their bum cheeks and trying not to scream).

I reached the toilet at the breakfast area and had the most painful, loud and hideous toilet experience I think I've ever had.

Sincere apologies if you are reading this book while eating. I hope I haven't put you off your food too much!

The jet lag, the water (however careful with water you are while abroad, sometimes the fruit can be washed in it), the time difference, the food and perhaps a little bit of food poisoning culminated in this wonderful, memorable experience.

And to top it off, this IBS flare-up lasted for ALL four days of our stay at this elegant hotel, which I'd been looking forward to for months.

Trust IBS to bring me right back down to reality, eh?

Back then – being far less organised than I would be now – I had no remedies with me, so I had to wait it out, while staying hydrated and trying to eat very plain foods.

What's the saying – fail to prepare and prepare to fail.

Or at least that's what I took from THAT experience anyway. These days, I plan ahead and consult my ultimate checklist whenever travelling to ensure no further trip is ruined (or at least disrupted) in quite the same way.

So for all those of you who have also caught the travel bug and want to make sure IBS doesn't get in your way of adventuring. Here goes…

BEFORE YOU TRAVEL

• Ensure all your medication is ready to pack, your prescriptions up to date and you take any over-the-counter remedies you might need.

• Call ahead to check the bathroom arrangements of your accommodation (or consult TripAdvisor).

• Call ahead at any hotels, restaurants and places of interest you might be visiting. TripAdvisor offers a search function where you can search for specific terms (i.e. vegan, dairy-free) on the page for each destination, which can be really helpful.

• Make sure you have plenty of IBS friendly snacks to hand.

• Make sure you have all of your vaccinations in place for your destination of choice.

• Let your travel companion know about your IBS (if you haven't already). Having someone you can confide in really helps, as having to keep your IBS 'under wraps' is another stress you don't need.

Packing

- UNDERWEAR (FOR SOME REASON, I'LL ALWAYS PACK DOUBLE THE AMOUNT I ACTUALLY NEED. DESPITE BEING TOILET TRAINED FOR OVER 23 YEARS NOW, WHEN IT COMES TO TRAVEL, I SEEM TO SEVERELY UNDERESTIMATE MY OWN ABILITY TO CONTROL MY BLADDER – OOPS).

- FLIP-FLOPS FOR HOT WEATHER OR WALKING BOOTS FOR AN OUTDOOR TRIP

- TRAINERS

- SOCKS

- T-SHIRTS

- TROUSERS OR SKIRTS

- DRESSES

- EVENING WEAR

- EVENING SHOES

- EXTRA UNDERWEAR (CONSULT POINT ABOVE, IN CASE YOU NEED A REASON WHY)

- HERBAL TEA (I ALWAYS GO FOR PEPPERMINT)

- A GOOD BOOK (TO TAKE YOUR MIND OFF THINGS OR KEEP YOU OCCUPIED IF YOU ARE CONFINED TO THE TOILET FOR ANY REASON)

- O HEAT PADS (THEY ARE USUALLY SOLD AS HEAT WARMERS FOR SHOULDER/BACK PAIN BUT YOU CAN GET THEM IN MOST CHEMISTS. THEY ESSENTIALLY ARE FLAT STICKY PADS THAT WARM UP WHEN THEY TOUCH YOUR SKIN. THEY ARE LIFE SAVERS FOR THE PLANE WHEN YOU CAN'T GET TO A HOT WATER BOTTLE OR A MICROWAVE)

- O EMPTY HOT WATER BOTTLE OR WHEAT BAG

- O IBS FRIENDLY SNACKS

- O A LIGHT JACKET (I AM FREEZING 99% OF THE TIME)

- O TOILETRIES

- O TOILET ROLL

- O WET WIPES

- O HAND SANITIZER

Travel Documents

- O PASSPORT

- O BOARDING PASSES

- O INSURANCE

- O HOTEL INFORMATION (WRITTEN IN LOCAL LANGUAGE)

- O GUIDEBOOK

Supplements

o   PROBIOTICS (I TAKE THESE DAILY AND WOULD
    SAY THEY ARE EVEN MORE IMPORTANT WHILE
    TRAVELLING, AS YOU ARE INTRODUCED TO NEW
    FOODS ETC)

o   PEPPERMINT OIL TABLETS (THESE CAN REALLY
    HELP TO SOOTHE AN IRRITATED DIGESTIVE
    SYSTEM)

o   IMODIUM (JUST IN CASE A THAILAND LIZARD
    DISASTER STRIKES)

o   LAXATIVES (TRAVEL CAN SOMETIMES CAUSE
    MY DIGESTIVE SYSTEM TO BUNG ITSELF UP,
    AND TRAVEL IS NO FUN IF YOU'RE SEVERELY
    CONSTIPATED. I PREFER THE NATURAL VARIETY,
    LIKE SENOKOT OR HOLLAND & BARRETT FRUIT &
    FIBRE CHEWABLES)

o   PILLBOXES (I ORGANISE MINE IN A WEEKLY
    PILLBOX SO THAT I KNOW WHAT I'VE TAKEN EACH
    DAY AND CAN CARRY THEM WITH ME ON A DAILY
    BASIS)

o   ANY OTHER MEDICATION YOU FIND HELPFUL

TIPS

Call ahead

I've been caught short on a couple of occasions where I've arrived at a hotel only to discover the gorgeous and luxurious bathroom is made entirely of glass, offering a beautiful view into the bedroom, but offering zero privacy when sharing with your travel companion. Ring your hotel ahead of your trip to check the bathroom arrangements as this can be a great way of putting your mind at rest, especially if it's a business trip where you might have to share with a colleague. Make sure you're going to feel as comfortable as possible and reassured in your upcoming arrangements.

Carry an IBS SOS kit with you at all times

Mine is small enough to fit into my handbag, but it essentially includes my supplements (activated charcoal is a great one, as are digestive enzymes), your hotel information written in a local language (should you get lost), your insurance, a bottle of filtered water, wet wipes, hand sanitizer and a spare change of underwear. Having that bag on you means you can relax knowing you're prepared for every eventuality!

Probiotics

Probiotics can be great at restoring the gut equilibrium, which is often interfered with by travel (different food, drinking water, air pressure, sporadic eating patterns). I use Alflorex and Just For Tummies, which are great for travelling as they don't need to be kept refrigerated and can be taken at any time of the day, with or without food.

Carry an IBS-friendly snack

Make sure you always carry an IBS-friendly snack with you, as airplane food and local restaurants aren't always great at fulfilling special requests. You can book a special meal on your flight, but make sure you do this at least 48 hours in advance, or you run the risk of them not being able to prepare for you.

Pack different options

Pack a variety of clothing options that you know you'll be comfortable in whether or not your stomach is playing up. I always overpack because I'd prefer to have extra than be caught short. Pack for appearance, for weather and for comfort!

Bring laxatives or Imodium

Depending on whether you're IBS-C, IBS-D or a combination of both, bring laxatives or Imodium tablets with you, just for reassurance. I often find that different food and eating patterns can cause horrible constipation, so I prepare for this by taking something to help keep my digestion regular even in unfamiliar surroundings.

Maintain your routine

Try and maintain a normal routine while you're away, just as when you're at home, as this will help to keep your IBS in check. If you normally have a peppermint tea after meals to ease your digestion, make sure you bring enough teabags away with you to carry on your routine.

Be prepared

Learn how to say what your intolerances are in the local language. Arrive prepared with phrases that will help you to express what foods you should avoid when you're eating out. You could even get a couple of cards printed (Vistaprint offer a free or very inexpensive service) with your intolerances written out in the local language. Simply hand them a card upon arrival so that they know what you can and can't eat.

Give yourself time

If you're planning the itinerary, make sure you leave enough time for toilet breaks and relaxing! A weekend break seems like fun, but if you're trying to cover all of the main attractions in a short space of time, that can be rather stressful in itself. Pick a few things to explore – and give yourself time in between each of them to enjoy the sights and recoup!

But above all, remember that you're there to have fun and explore this exciting new destination.

Travel is an incredible tool to relax the mind and take you on an adventure – so your IBS doesn't have to interfere.

To prove how far I've come from the European travel disaster with the previous boyfriend (refer back to the dating chapter for a recap on that marvellous tale), I actually went camping for a week in America last year – with a bunch of strangers.

We spent the night in the gorgeous National Parks at the Grand Canyon, Yosemite and in Arizona, enjoying incredible scenery and making our dinner around a campfire. And, of course, this incredibly beautiful experience was also accompanied by having to deal with camping toilets which were a few minutes' walk away – in the pitch black dark.

So if I can manage it, you can too! Although I'm not saying camping is a necessity, your own bathroom is obviously always preferable - let's face it!

One thing I also find really tricky when travelling is getting used to a 'new toilet'. It sounds absolutely ridiculous if you've never experienced this before – a toilet is just a toilet, right? But when you suffer from IBS, things like your OWN toilet become a comfort blanket and it feels strange and scary to have to 'go' somewhere new.

CBT and retraining my cognitive thought processes surrounding this topic has been the most effective way of treating and dealing with this issue. However, it definitely still crops up now and again, especially if I'm having to share bathrooms with friends or even my boyfriend.

My boyfriend and I are lucky to travel the world a lot together with my job and we stay in some absolutely gorgeous hotels, but as mentioned above, the bathrooms aren't always the most accommodating for those with digestive troubles. They certainly haven't been designed by someone who has had IBS, that's for sure!

One such wonderful experience was when the toilet cubicle at one hotel was made entirely out of GLASS. A fabulous invention if you've ever had a penchant for watching your travel companion take a midnight wee but also hugely frustrating privacy-wise, especially if you – like me – often have to spend a fair amount of time huddled on the loo, straining, mopping up and looking generally not-quite-my-best-self. It's certainly one way to kill any kind of romance after a big meal, that's for sure!

The best way of dealing with this is to be totally honest and frank with your travel companion. Let's face it, in a glass cubicle, there is NOWHERE to hide so there's no point even trying to keep things to yourself.

One thing I do regularly with my boyfriend is to ask him to go for a wander around the hotel whenever I 'need to go' or plonk him on the balcony with a book. It sounds pretty hilarious but it works and I feel so much more comfortable knowing I have a teeny bit more privacy.

Also, if you're a hotelier wondering how to accommodate IBS-ers, hit me up! I have a huge list of pointers – one is a 'music switch' for the bathroom, so you can pop on some rock or classical to muffle any marvellous bathroom sounds.

If you're going on a city break or hiking holiday (I'm afraid to say, you WON'T find me on the latter, I'm not a hiking kinda gal, but I have tried it in the past), then you will have to deal with the perils that are PUBLIC toilets, and boy oh boy, do I love them. Especially in the US, where for some very bizarre reason, toilet doors aren't made to fit the cubicle. So every experience usually involves you being able to see a slither of whatever is happening outside of your cubicle, usually the backs of people's heads while they are washing their hands.

But it has also resulted in probably the single most awkward experience of my entire life, when I maintained eye contact with a very nosey lady while I was going to the loo. I didn't want to break eye contact, nor did she. It was very unnerving and I now totally appreciate the privacy of UK toilets, whereby the door is made to fit the cubicle and offers up a larger degree of one's own pooping and peeing space. Phew!

I've always referred to women who exercise while they are on their period as 'those who were going to survive the apocalypse' because let's face it, when you're in pain, the LAST thing you want to do is pound the treadmill.

CHAPTER 9

Gentle Exercise

I've always referred to women who exercise while they are on their period as 'those who were going to survive the apocalypse' because let's face it, when you're in pain, the LAST thing you want to do is pound the treadmill.

I've never been big on exercise or physical activity of any kind.

I vaguely remember winning an egg and spoon race aged 6 one year, only because everyone else dropped theirs. The only race I ever won.

Slow and steady wins the race, and I came out on top!

In school, I was ALWAYS picked last on sports day and somehow ended up being lumped with activities no-one else wanted to do. One year, I had to represent our class in the javelin, despite not actually knowing what on earth competing in it actually entailed. I was first up to compete and almost immediately it was clear that I'd got it confused with the high jump. I will say no more.

But anyway, what I'm trying to say is exercise was NEVER on my radar when I was first diagnosed with IBS.

My parents used to gently coax me into staying more active, as a means of easing up my symptoms. But I didn't listen. There was NO way I wanted to be caught short running on a field while being struck by an IBS 'urge to go'.

But as I've grown up and my symptoms have developed somewhat, I've found gentle exercise to be a really effective way of managing stress, constipation and trapped wind.

Keeping your body moving can encourage your digestion to start moving too, which if you had bouts of serious constipation like I did, is definitely a good thing.

Similarly, if you're more prone to diarrhoea and bloating, a session where you're moving your body can release any trapped air and gas. In fact, it might work so well that the trapped air and gas may come out during a very quiet, candle-lit yoga class. I will say no more. Nope, I'm definitely not speaking from experience.

Weaving in some gentle exercise into your daily routine is beneficial for IBS in many ways, but it's also great for the mind too. As I work for myself, from home, I'm often stuck indoors all day and I don't interact with the world like the average person might. Don't get me wrong, I totally love my own company and I'm quite content spending time by myself, but I NEED to move, get out the house or do some form of physical activity at least once per day or I find my mental health can take a dive.

For me, my solution involves having a couple of different go-tos, depending on how my symptoms are at any one time. If I'm symptom-free, I'm quite happy to go to the gym, go to a class or venture outside for a walk.

If I am feeling more run down and symptomatic, then I will choose to do a workout at home. YouTube is a fantastic source of inspiration for workout routines as you can usually find something that will accommodate your ability, location and time.

One of my favourite workouts is the 7-minute workout by Lucy Wyndam-Read. It features 7 simple exercises that you do for 60 seconds each. If I am feeling quite poorly, I'll try and do just this once per day (it is only seven minutes of your time anyway, so there's no excuse why you can't fit it in) and for any more dynamic movements, I'll tone it down a little bit.

If I'm suffering VERY severely with symptoms then I'll try something different altogether, which is very slow gentle stretching to coax out trapped wind, relieve pain and relax my mind. Think of it like a sloth doing yoga. Slowly, slowly.

And speaking of yoga, I went on a four-day yoga retreat in the beautiful Spanish mountains of Granada last year. I didn't quite know what to expect, but I was going through a really tough time mentally and I could sense it was starting to have an impact on my IBS symptoms flaring up again.

So the offer to visit (a blog opportunity) came at exactly the right time. Despite being initially cynical about whether I was a 'yoga' person, I took so much away from the experience that I want to make it a yearly thing. Something I do for myself and my mind, as a preventative measure to stop my IBS symptoms kicking up a fuss.

I actually wrote an article on my blog about my experience there and I wanted to include it in this book because it describes my exact feelings and thoughts at the time, and regurgitating my original thoughts wouldn't do it justice.

Many of the things are relevant to IBS sufferers in terms of de-stressing, retuning the mind and focusing our attention on US, rather than the stresses, strains and bustle of every-day life. Our body is the only place we'll ever live, so it's vital to take care of it.

SO HERE ARE 6 SURPRISING THINGS I LEARNED ON A YOGA RETREAT...

Friends and family will know what a cynical person I am.

I tend to write things off before I've even tried them, which is probably testament to both my cynicism and my stubbornness.

And so, for the above reasons, I firmly decided around the age of 18, that I just wasn't a 'yoga' person.

I'm highly strung, my mind is constantly whirring with ideas and I have a phobia of toe socks.

You know, those strange material creatures that frequent yoga classes *(or at least the ones I'd tried previously)* that provide a space for each individual toe to hibernate.

They creeped me out. They still do. I won't lie.

Anyway, with all of the above considered, it may come as a surprise for you to know that last month, I embarked on my first EVER yoga retreat. With Kaliyoga. In the sunny mountains of Spain.

I accepted the invitation because at the time it arrived in my inbox, I was in a flurry of panic (having had three panic attacks in one week) and I was what you'd probably describe (in true millennial manner) 'burnt out'.

With eight other bloggers in tow, we flew to Malaga airport for four days of the kind of relaxation that was previously alien to me.

And upon returning, I think I've been converted.

You won't ever find me wearing toe socks. SOZ. But I learned so much from this special trip that I wanted to share it with you.

So sit, back, grab a cup of tea, *take off them bleedin' toe socks* and read on...

We all need ME time

And I'm not just talking about a hot bath here and there.

We need proper 'ME' time, long enough to feel comfortable in our own company and in our own mind.

Long enough to gather together what's been on your mind and work through it.

Not just pampering me time, but perhaps slightly uncomfortable – at first – me time, that heals us from the inside, out.

And Kaliyoga's gorgeous surroundings was the perfect place to indulge in a bit of me time.

Nestled away in the gorgeous mountains of Grenada, the nearest town is accessible by car but far enough away that the only sounds in the air are the gentle hum of wildlife and the twinkling chimes of the gorgeous farmhouse's terrace.

Guests stay in beautiful bedrooms in the main house, in casita cabins outdoors (I stayed in a stunning pastel blue one overlooking the pool) or in the summer, in tepees.

Your days are occupied by morning and evening sessions at the Yogashala, hikes in the mountains, reading your book by the pool and other added extras, such as reflexology, sound healing or Thai massages – that you can add on depending on your preferences.

This sense of freedom and relaxation really helps you adjust your focus and renew your energy.

I found it immensely helpful in having the time to visualise what I REALLY want out of life. And what really matters to me.

This realisation has since instilled me with some innate sense of calm that sweeps over me whenever I sense that I'm starting to panic.

We were taught to visualise our thoughts coming and going in our mind like the tide. The waves sweeping in and out, whispering gently through our body and leaving calmly in the same way they arrived.

This has REALLY helped me to stop, take a breath and calm down whenever I sense I'm starting to fall into panic mode.

We need to disconnect

It's 2018 and rightly or wrongly, our smartphones know everything about us. They are pretty much surgically attached to our hands and they contain our memories, organise our daily routines and even track how many steps we take.

They have given us immense amounts of freedom *(we can travel anywhere in the world and get around even with a language barrier)* and they connect us to the outside world, without us even having to leave our homes.

But while they do have amazing benefits in keeping us connected, we do need to remember that we don't always NEED to be connected to everyone else.

It's healthy to disconnect and detox from the digital world once in a while and luckily, Kaliyoga gave us the opportunity to do this.

Obviously, we did venture online a few times for work purposes, but most of the time - we re-learned to just enjoy being in the moment, chatting with one another face-to-face, rather than behind a screen.

And when you start to rely on your smartphone less, strange things start to happen.

You see the things you don't usually see because you're distracted.

Your mind wanders less and you live a little more presently.

You feel a little less cluttered and a touch more 'free'.

You slow down, care a little less about what's going on in other people's lives and figure out what you want from yours.

I'd highly recommend it.

The right food fuels the mind

In the past few years, I've become much more aware of what it is that I'm putting into my body.

I have been plagued by horrible IBS symptoms since the age of 14 and changing up my diet was the only real way to get a handle on things.

But certain issues still persisted. I was tired all the time, lethargic, low energy and at the time – sorry David – very grouchy.

I did wonder whether what I was eating was playing a part, but it wasn't until I spent time at Kaliyoga that I truly realised how big an impact food was having.

The food at the yoga retreat might sound daunting for some – with no meat, processed sugar, gluten, dairy or alcohol on the menu, and many dishes 'raw'. However, for me, I was excited and intrigued to see if it was the answer I'd been looking for.

Because just a day or so in, I was already feeling better within myself. I awoke in the morning without wanting to groan in horror at having to start the day with low energy.

The raw dishes were extremely tasty, wholesome and filling. And there was something really lovely about knowing that everything you were putting into your body was doing good. It was nutritious and delicious!

I was especially impressed by the three-course evening meal, which allowed us to experiment with new flavours and really inspire our own meal plans back home.

And talking of home, if you do miss the food upon arriving back (which invariably, you will – it's incredible – for lack of a better word), then you might want to treat yourself to a Kaliyoga cookbook – featuring recipes that have taken years to tweak and construct by the team in Spain (they wanted to make sure it was perfect), but that you'll want to cook up as soon as you get home.

Affirmations may sound cringeworthy but they are so powerful

I'd never quite appreciated how powerful affirmations can be, until I started saying them daily.

Following a sound healing session with Kim (*which you can hear more about in my vlog of this trip - it was quite an experience*), she recommended I repeat three individualised affirmations on a daily basis, for forty days straight.

I won't go into detail about what mine were, as they will be different for everyone – but essentially, they are three or so 'I AMs' that aim to conquer something you're feeling or going through.

For example, this could be a mix of 'I am confident', 'I am independent', 'I am a strong', 'I am doing my best', 'I am beautiful'. You get the idea.

Words have immense power in changing your mindset, your goals and your drive.

Try it for a few days, stand in front of the mirror and repeat your chosen affirmations either out loud or in your head. And see what a difference it can make.

At first, it feels a bit silly, but the more you say it, the more they start to make an impact.

Innately, I think we have something engrained inside of us that when we look in the mirror, we are drawn to the negatives.

It only takes you changing your mindset to change this.

Yoga isn't a competition

I know in parts of London and for some yoga classes I've been to previously, there's a certain snobbery around yoga.

If you're a beginner, you stick out like a sore thumb and it can be quite embarrassing.

Especially because in situations where everyone is serious and breathing in time with one another, I just get the urge to giggle.

It happens uncontrollably and this only makes the situation EVEN more embarrassing.

In my past (basic) experience with yoga, it's always felt very competitive and very 'us and them', if you're a novice.

Kaliyoga completely wiped the slate clean when it came to this mentality and proved that yoga isn't a competition.

It's about learning to relax, unwind, restore your mind and connect with yourself.

The yoga they practise is very slow, perfect for all abilities and can be taken at your own pace.

There's no sniggering or sneering looks if you fall on your bum (thank goodness, because it happened to me a lot) and it feels more like a mindfulness session than a sport.

Which I love.

Because I was training my core and my mind.

The main farmhouse is a restored family home and you're told upon arrival to treat the place as your own home for the week too.

The lounge is filled with chatter in the evenings, with an evening 'mocktail' to wrap up the day and a sense of belonging.

I'm not sure quite how they've created such a warm, friendly and inclusive environment so organically, but they've just got it SO right.

The only validation we need is our own

The digital world has created a new dopamine release that we get from pleasure-seeking or validation-seeking, especially for those who spent a lot of time on social media.

This dopamine release is addictive and when we don't have it – or have too much of it – studies have shown it can actually be anxiety inducing.

This all sounds rather scary and technical but when we think about it, it's true.

We get a small 'high' when someone likes our photo, validates us, our content, our work and our outfit.

But over time, we need more and more of that validation in order to get the same 'high'.

This can, in turn, make us feel pressure, or even present itself as anxious feelings. I know in my case it has.

It sounds really silly, but when it's something engrained into our everyday lives, we can't help but get affected by it. Especially in bloggers cases, where it's sometimes their full-time jobs.

And so one final thing that the Kaliyoga trip taught me was that the only real validation we need is our own.

We shouldn't be relying upon the validation of others to be happy, because that puts the power of happiness into someone else's hands.

True confidence is knowing that you alone are enough!

Now I know a yoga retreat isn't everyone's cup of tea (mind you, I didn't think it was mine – and it was) nor is it even feasible for everyone – with a family, commitments and financial constraints, but many of the points above can be easily put into the context of any situation. Me time, medi-tation, regular exercise and yoga – hey, if you can't get out of the house to do yoga – there are plenty of YouTube classes you could do from the comfort of your bedroom.

Above all, you need to look after yourself. Exercise the body and the mind simultaneously and remember that you are worth investing in.

WORDS HAVE IMMENSE POWER IN

CHANGING YOUR MINDSET, YOUR

GOALS AND YOUR DRIVE.

Maintaining balance in your life – between work life, home life and your social life – is a pretty difficult couple of plates to juggle all at once for the average person.

But throw IBS into the mix and you have another wobbly, fragile plate to spin.

CHAPTER 10

Social Life

Over the years, I'd say out of everything – my social life is the one thing I've never been quite able to master and I've lost a LOT of friends in the process.

To put things into context, I have only started being open about my IBS struggles publicly in the last 4-5 years, so prior to that my bouts of illness and cancelling last minute, probably appeared flaky and unreliable – so I don't really blame any friendships that suffered as a result.

However, since I started sharing my story with IBS and talking about digestive health on the internet, everyone seems to have their very own opinion on my bowels.

And whether or not a friend truly decides to understand and empathise with what it is I'm going through is key to whether a friendship will survive.

It's strangely therapeutic that everyone knows my digestive system has issues, because I no longer feel I'm suffering in silence and treading carefully as so not to reveal my 'big' secret.

Friends now talk openly about their poo dilemmas with me and we REALLY contribute to breaking down the stigma associated with the poo taboo, purely because we are so TMI.

But it's also frustrating because many people inside (and outside) your circle have opinions on your bowels too. I've had plenty of pearls of unsolicited advice and strange responses over the years, which I thought I'd provide some examples of below:

"My father's uncle's brother's cousin's sister's friend's dog has IBS… It turns out she was lactose intolerant. Maybe that's your issue?"

"Yeah, I've had a bad stomach recently too. Mine has been SOOOO painful"

"I remember back in 1986, I had terrible wind and diarrhoea"

"I had IBS once, so I know how you feel. But mine was MUCH worse"

"You look okay to me. Just suck it up, you'll be fine"

"So, what CAN YOU actually eat then?"

"You just need to eat healthier and exercise more"

"Ew, that's so gross"

"I don't believe in all that rubbish."

"It's all in your head"

"But I thought you were better. Why are you ill again?"

"But one bite won't hurt you. Why don't you just try it?"

"Ooh it looks like someone is being a very fussy eater"

I appreciate the sentiment of trying to be helpful and none of the above things said to me have been said in malice. I know sometimes people have default reactions or statements that they use if they don't know what else to say. As human beings, we want to offer advice and try to help – and sometimes the right intention is there but the delivery is off. So it's important to give people the benefit of the doubt and encourage them to ask questions, be inquisitive and learn more – rather than making snap judgements.

Admittedly, it's difficult to know the right thing to say to someone who suffers from IBS, because from an outsider's perspective it can be frustrating to not know how to help. I remember my mum being in tears because she felt powerless to help me. It can be tricky to know what will be the most beneficial thing to say.

But please rest assured friends, sometimes I and others like me just need a sympathetic ear (and perhaps a toilet close by). Your support alone means more than you know.

The wonderful thing about invisible conditions like IBS is that I probably do look fine on the outside. And I suppose it's a compliment that I look like my normal self when there's so much inner turmoil going on. But if someone had a broken leg, people generally wouldn't tell them to suck it up and walk on it. Just because IBS can't be seen it doesn't mean it's not there.

And I get it, tough love is needed sometimes, but an IBS sufferer can already feel hideously guilty for 'over-reacting' about their symptoms, or letting their symptoms take over their life. If it wasn't worth moaning about, we probably wouldn't be moaning.

A default reaction in humans is to snap back with a response they think might be helpful such as '*don't worry*'. It has kind intention, but rarely provides any desired positive effect on the recipient. In fact, it can leave us feeling like the other person is flippantly ignoring what we are going through or doesn't feel like our worries or anxieties are valid. The best thing you can do to someone who is going through something like IBS is to listen to their worries. Give them an open arena to air their concerns and feel privileged that they have chosen you to open up to. Listen, give them a hug (if appropriate) and let them know you are there for them. Try to empathise with them and let them know that you are on their team.

There's no winning formula when it comes to friendships because each friend adds something different to your life.

I'm certainly not the friendship guru, but to me, a friendship is a two-sided thing.

It takes two to tango, and all that.

Just like a relationship, a friendship should bring something to the table.

We have different friends for different reasons.

You'll have Sarah, who is a complete hoot and can make you cry and laugh within minutes of seeing her, you'll have Sally, who knows everything about everyone and fills you in on all the things you don't pick up on, you'll have Susan from work, who reciprocates your eye rolls in meetings and is there to share work woes over a sandwich with you.

Then you'll have Barbara, who is your go-to for advice, Beatrice, who is your ultimate organised travel buddy, and then Bella, who shares your love of music and inspires you to venture off to gigs and festivals.

And you might even have friends whose names don't ALL begin with the same letter.

But you never know, I had three friends at school called Charlotte.

Anyway, my point is – a good friend doesn't necessarily have to fit into set criteria, but they do have to add to your life in some way. However small or huge that 'way' may be.

A good friend may be initially irritated that you've cancelled your lunch together, but they'll understand.

And like dating, IBS can be a good buffer for figuring out the people you want to invest your time, energy and love into.

DON'T SAY YES TO EVERYTHING

Often we say 'yes' to every invitation, every lunch-date and every social get-together because we feel it's easier than saying no. Deep down, we know that we're eventually going to have to cancel later down the line, but it's easier to say yes initially for fear of upsetting the person or being excluded from future invites.

Previously, I would always agree to a plan, knowing full well I'd be uncomfortable in the situation. I'd then worry for weeks about the social engagement. I'd upset my stomach in the process (because of the anxiety) and I'd then let them down at the last minute because invariably my stomach would be in turmoil. This unhelpful situation I'd created was purely because I wasn't brave enough to just say NO (thank you) at the very beginning. I could have eliminated so much worry and upset if I'd have just been honest in the first place.

Nowadays, I don't say yes to things (nor do I suggest things) unless I have every intention of being there. Obviously, sometimes things happen that we can't help – like the time I was supposed to be on a Thames Afternoon Tea River Cruise with five friends, but that morning I couldn't leave the bathroom because I had painful diarrhoea, but when you cancel LESS, people no longer assume you're just being a flake.

BE OPEN AND HONEST

This is a pretty obvious one and follows the same guidance I've given in other chapters, so I won't go into too much detail, but in essence, be honest with friends. Confide in people you trust and enjoy the reassurance that you have someone 'on your team'.

Don't feel you have to hide or suffer in silence. Invisible illnesses can be tricky enough without feeling you're alone. Often, you may find that confiding in someone else allows them to open up too. I've discovered a few friends who have

IBS too, which can be unbelievably helpful as you can be sure that someone knows what you're going through.

SUGGEST IBS-FRIENDLY ACTIVITIES

If you'd still love the company that social endeavours provide, but you're worried about the usual social situation not accommodating the worst-case IBS scenario, then don't be afraid to suggest things that are going to work best for you.

For me, it's awkward and quiet situations that I worry about the most. So I always suggest meeting somewhere busy and loud, with plenty of distractions to help me feel as comfortable as possible.

I often find it very difficult staying at other people's houses because there are so many factors that can provide difficulty – food, bathroom situations, sleeping arrangements and not having my home comforts (like my hot water bottle, or my bed) if I have a slight flare-up. So I always make sure to extend an offer to friends to stay at our house. I love being the hostess because it means that I can be around friends, but still be in the environment I'm most comfortable in. There's always a way around a situation if you genuinely WANT to partake in it.

WHAT SALLY SAYS ABOUT SANDRA SAYS MORE ABOUT SALLY THAN SANDRA

I've been at the receiving end of a few bitchy remarks in my time. I've been called gross, I've been spoken about behind my back (and it's invariably got back to me) and I've even been laughed at. It really upset me at the time. And, of course, in true IBS style, even caused a flare-up. But as I've got older, I realised that people's reactions say far more about them, than they do about me. Usually, it's a sign of immaturity and insecurity on their part and it takes a lot of strength on your part not to take it personally. I've found that the best way to respond to these comments is in a kind way because unleashing anger or upset can actually make you feel worse. To the person that felt the need to talk about me behind my back and make fun of my chronic illness, I'm so sorry you felt the need to do this. Behind the exterior shell, we all have hardships going on and at some point in our futures, we are all going to need a bit of love and empathy. So right now, I'm sending you yours.

TO THE PERSON WHO IS UNSYMPATHETIC OR UNHELPFUL

Sometimes you'll encounter the odd friend who offers the truly unhelpful remark 'it's all in your head'. This is a particularly hurtful statement because it not only demeans what you're going through, but it's also ignorant to the feelings of the recipient of the comment. Indeed, I also think, 'oh it's just in my head,' as I plonk myself onto the toilet for the seventh time that morning. If only IBS was the myth they thought it was, eh!

It can be tempting to respond back emotionally, but usually this can burn a friendship unnecessarily. Some people do have different ways of looking at certain situations in life, depending on how they've been brought up or what they've been through in their own life. It doesn't mean they are a bad person or totally unsympathetic, it just means they have a different viewpoint than you. It is difficult to empathise with someone for something they don't understand. It's up to you (if you see fit) at this point to educate the person, ask them if they have any questions about your IBS and open up. It's important to keep the dialogue going, open up, communicate and never feel silenced or shut down. It's easier said than done, but no-one has the power to make you feel a certain way. The only person holding that power of feeling is you. That said, you are allowed to feel a bit miffed when someone has expressed something unsympathetic or unhelpful. I would be too, but use your experiences to educate others. And try not to take it personally.

UNDERSTAND THAT IBS CAN BE UNPREDICTABLE

I appreciate that for some friends, it can be frustrating when I look 'well' on the outside, but have to cancel plans at the last minute. So explain the unpredictability of your IBS and make friends aware of your situation, so that they understand that you value being open, trustworthy and reliable, but your symptoms can sometimes get in the way of upholding these values. Flexibility is key and the right friends will always understand.

I remember after my first IBS attack, I felt so angry at my body.

How dare it let me down so hideously? How could it betray me? I couldn't believe it.

This set about a negative spiral of self-punishment and hatred.

CHAPTER 11

Self-Love
(Cut yourself some slack)

You often hear of teenage girls hating their own body appearance-wise, but I felt let down for other reasons.

I felt out of control, confused and at a complete loss as to how I could deal with it.

I appreciate that I probably sounded like a complete moaning myrtle at times. There were (and are) people in the world dying of awful diseases. People getting a cancer diagnosis or ending up in terrible accidents and never seeing their loved ones ever again. I was constantly aware of how minor my symptoms were in the grand scheme of things. But as much as I tried to look at the positives and tell myself I should appreciate the fact that my syndrome wasn't going to kill me, I did let them get the better of me at times.

But being kind to yourself is key to getting better. You have to set those feelings of disgust, frustration, self-doubt, self-punishment and negativity free and learn to love yourself – IBS and all.

Interestingly, a couple of years ago, I conducted interviews as part of my university degree with many psychologists, gut experts and gastroenterologists.

Many of the experts I spoke to had looked into the psychological aspects of bowel conditions and believed that even though the symptoms can be very embarrassing, the answer to overcoming them is not in the hands of other people, but the sufferers themselves.

The overriding consensus was that we often fear the disapproval of others, so we create feelings of shame and disgust that we project onto others even though they may not have a problem with it. The stigma is often greater in OUR mind rather than outside of it.

Having a heightened awareness of other people's perceptions can be detrimental to living with bowel conditions on a daily basis.

When we feel stigmatised, it inevitably erodes our self-confidence. The key to breaking the cycle is to talk about the condition. It's important to develop feelings of self-confidence in order to defeat the embarrassment.

INVEST IN YOURSELF

It's important to invest in ourselves and feed our bodies with the right food, allow it to have the correct amount of rest and unwind from the stresses of daily life. In today's society, we are so focused on filling our every waking moment with a 'productive' activity that we forget to give ourselves space to actually BREATHE. So spend 15-20 minutes every day investing in something that positively feeds your wellbeing, whether it's listening to music you love, reading a novel that has been on the shelf for ages, writing or gardening. And be sure to choose uplifting music or reading material too – often reading the news or even the newspaper can have a negative effect on us as we often read about tragedies or things that may worry us.

SILENCE THE INNER CRITIC FROM TIME TO TIME

An inner critic can be a good thing, as it can motivate us and inspire us to do better. However, we also have to know when to silence the inner critic. We are often aware of how we treat others and are conscious that we should be kind, complimentary and polite with others, and yet we do not afford ourselves the same treatment. We wouldn't criticise our work colleague unkindly on a daily or hourly basis, so why do we subject ourselves to it? To start with, try to give yourself a compliment once a day at the very least. Learn to praise yourself and congratulate yourself – even for small victories! And then as time goes on, write down 1-3 things per week that you appreciate about yourself. Are you a good listener? Are you kind? Or maybe you make your bed every day? Whatever it is, whatever you appreciate about yourself, write it down in a specific notebook. Then at the end of the month, go through everything together. There's a lot lot more about yourself that you can appreciate and it sometimes helps to see it all written down on paper.

KEEP A DIARY

This may not be totally applicable to everyone, but writing is a huge therapeutic help to me. By spilling out my emotions from my mind onto paper, I feel a weight lifted from me instantly, as it helps me to make sense of bigger situations that can seem a little overwhelming at the time. Some of the most famous and admired people in history kept diaries to get them through arduous and difficult times – Anne Frank, Nelson Mandela, Virginia Woolf, to name a few. Often we detach ourselves from real life and rarely look at what we are going through as a 'bigger picture'. However, journaling and diary entries help us to re-engage with this. It helps us to manage our emotions, our feelings and potentially see things more clearly. Putting pen to paper can help you to unplug, reset and clear your emotional baggage.

BE YOUR OWN BEST FRIEND

Often, part of the key to self-love is acceptance and learning to love your own company. I've always been quite an introvert and I love my own company; however, even I have struggled to 'be my own best friend' and be totally comfortable doing things by myself, for myself. I've always worried far too deeply about what others would think about me being on my own. If I was dining at a restaurant, would they think I'd been stood up by a date? If I was at the cinema alone, would they think that I had no friends? In reality, no-one is really analysing us in this much depth, they are too concerned with their own lives. And if they were thinking that, then it is probably a reflection of their own thoughts and fears about being spotted alone.

HAVE A SLOGAN OR A PERSONAL MANTRA

Nike, McDonalds and L'Oréal all have their very own tag-lines, so why can't you? Often it helps to have a mantra to repeat to ourselves whenever we need a pick me up or a lift of positivity. It sounds ridiculous but can be really helpful in engraining positive messages into our minds, rather than negative ones. A personal mantra is essentially a one-line affirmation to motivate you and uplift your mind, to encourage you to keep pushing forward and going after what it is you want. Maybe yours could be:

'I can't control what others think, just how I react' – remind yourself that it's a total waste of energy to worry about the views of others, which you cannot control. Your reactions, actions and motivations are all that matter.

'Everything we want to be, can be and will be is inside us right now' – this is an affirmation that reminds you that you hold the key to shaping your future and have the potential to reach for whatever it is in life you desire. It's inside you already, you just have to find where it's located.

'Don't let what you can't do, interfere with what you can do' – so often in life we focus on what we may be restricted from doing, rather than what we CAN do. Focus on these can do's – and do them as best you can.

'All I can do is my best' – this was a huge one for me in school because I put a surmounting pressure on myself to achieve high grades and impress my teachers and parents. I would constantly compare myself to others around me and study as hard as I could. I would be so anxious before exams (despite all my preparation) so this simple affirmation would help to reassure me that all I could do is my best. That's all anyone (myself or otherwise) could ever ask for.

'I am enough' – in the past few years, I've had some huge life lessons and learning curves that taught me an awful lot. I have a thicker skin and a brighter smile as a result. I've learned to forgive, to be strong, to dream and to believe in myself. It all sounds ridiculously cliched I know, but if you'd have told me several years ago where I'd be now, I'd have probably laughed in your face. Throughout my teenage years and early twenties, there was always a little voice in my head (the infamous inner critic) that said I wasn't quite enough. Pretty enough, smart enough, tough enough, confident enough, bold enough, social enough, loud enough, charismatic enough. But I've learned that I am enough. As I am. Before, I'd have put down any of my successes to 'luck', but I've realised it's not about luck. Instead, it's credit to my hard work, passion and efforts. Make sure that you know you are enough, too.

At the very end of the book, I have included my 9 'rules of life', in which you'll find the personal mantra that I use now. See if you can find it!

One thing that helped me massively in coming to terms with IBS and the issues that it presents was, of course, to talk about it.

And in doing so, I discovered that I wasn't alone with my symptoms.

There were other people too – friends, colleagues and peers, who had been through a similar experience with digestive discomfort – some of whom had been suffering at the same time, but we were both too scared to speak up.

CHAPTER 12

Case Studies

truly do believe that the key to unlocking the 'stigma' associated with the 'poo taboo' is to keep an open, honest and frank dialogue about IBS going. There is no shame, no embarrassment and no need to feel alone.

As a means of illustrating this, I wanted to dedicate an entire chapter to featuring some other wonderful people who have also been brave enough to share their journey with IBS online. Because 'taming the tummy' isn't JUST about my story, it's about YOURS.

"I first started experiencing health issues in 2014. I did a bit of my own research (hello, doctor Google) and thought it might be a dairy allergy. I cut it out for a couple of weeks and felt WAY better, so I decided to take my evidence to the doctors and ask them to confirm it. In the end, it was established that I had a dairy allergy and whilst I was having allergy tests, they discovered a problem with gluten, pork, barley, beef; basically, all of these 'trigger' foods typical for IBS sufferers.

I was told when I got these results that I had IBS and my symptoms would lessen if I could adhere to the low FODMAP diet and eliminate the foods that caused me problems. I remember leaving the doctor's office and calling my mum and sobbing, "I'm never going to have a wedding cake!!" Why was that my first thought?!

It was a really hard time, to be honest, but I did my best to remain positive and see my new diet as a challenge and something that I should at least try to make fun. I never thought I'd be able to keep it up, but I started feeling better so soon that I realised I'd rather have a life without gluten and dairy if it meant I'd feel better. Sure, I had a little ceremony to mourn the pizzas I would no longer be able to eat, but apart from that, I was pretty brave about the whole thing.

I suffer from anxiety anyway and the connection between the two conditions is incredibly frustrating for a couple of reasons. In part, because people are very quick to tell you that a lot of your IBS symptoms are 'all in your head' and in part, because the illness IS so stressful that you do start to feel worse the minute you stress about it. When I'm having a bad flare-up, even now, it really takes its toll on my mental health; my boyfriend very often comes home to me lying on the sofa with a huge stomach and an utterly miserable attitude! It's hard to stay positive when you're ill!

In the early days of my IBS diagnosis, I found it incredibly stressful; I'd scour menus and get really embarrassed when I had to make a big deal out of ordering and making sure the waiter knew I wasn't just on a 'fad diet'. I also HATED the idea of going out when I was having a flare-up because I was bloated and I felt rubbish, but mostly because I didn't want to spend all night holding in farts! (Do you know how many times I have to pretend to go outside for fresh air when actually I just want to have a little trump!?)

Even now, nearly five years on, I still hate staying at other people's houses. This is not only because I like to be near my own bathroom, but also because I hate being a pain for anyone cooking and I unfortunately always will be. It has got a lot easier though and I've learned not to beat myself up! If I broke my leg, I wouldn't feel guilty arriving at a friend's house and not being able to get up the stairs, so why do I need to feel guilty for not being able to eat something? On a practical level, I very often take my own food with me when I go out; sometimes I'll precook a jacket potato and wrap it in tinfoil and put in my bag, sometimes I'll do the same with a chicken leg, and I am very rarely found without a Nakd bar or a packet of oatcakes in my bag. It's not always fun but at least that way you don't go hungry! Truthfully, it's been a bit of a nightmare.

Certainly, with my career, I am lucky to be self-employed and fortunate that a big part of my job is sharing my life (and often my IBS symptoms) but there have been days where my symptoms have been so severe that I have been unable to work. In January of this year, I had to take a week off as I just wasn't up to working. I find it very difficult when I look back at the month and see that I didn't earn anything for a whole week because I was unable to work! There have been countless days that I've lost to doctor's appointments or getting lost in supermarket aisles trying to find something to eat (kind of joking, kind of not!).

By nature I am not a 'sick' person, I hate getting back into bed and I very rarely don't work, so I do get really annoyed with my symptoms because they force me to be something that I don't like being at all! My boyfriend and I have been together for over six years which means he's been through all of this with me. When I eat something fatty or heavy or with a lot of sugar in, I get very farty and that's a bugger for romance! We'll very often go out for a romantic dinner and end up with me trumping in the bathroom whilst he lies in bed pretending not to hear. The LAST thing I want to do when I feel like this is to get intimate, and bless him, he really does understand! Sex and gas are not the one, not for me at any rate!

My advice would be simply to make the most of the time when you're not bloated. Feeling guilty when you get into bed doesn't help anyone and overthinking only makes it worse. If your partner is a decent person, they won't care AT ALL and only want you to be well. Spending time together in the mornings before you've eaten can be great and working out what works for you, even when you are experiencing a flare-up, is really helpful. You might not want to be in a seated position, for example, should your body mistakenly think you're sitting on the loo! So listen to your body. I was so brash and so ignorant with all of this at the beginning; I didn't see the connection between my head and my tummy, or between my surroundings and my symptoms. I realise now that when I'm stressed it gets worse and there are so many factors at play. If I'm in pain, I stop what I'm doing and take a rest. If I'm bloated, I try to be more diligent with my food. Don't beat yourself up for an illness out of your control and trust your body and its cravings because it's trying to do right by you! I have also found exercise to be a lifesaver, running in particular, mostly because I can fart on the go and there's no-one around to notice!"

"I can remember feeling very isolated because of my troublesome digestive symptoms. My main disturbance is bloating – I can often look about seven months pregnant! The bloating will start as soon as I eat or drink anything in the morning and it gets progressively more painful throughout the day, which invariably interrupts my social plans for the evening. I feel constantly nauseous, which impacts my appetite and I suffer from awful stomach aches and unrelenting cramps. My go-to antidote is usually a hot water bottle, a hot bath and a cup of peppermint tea! My symptoms have been ruling my life for the past year now and I was too embarrassed for a while to even tell my own mum about what was going on, despite me usually being totally open with her. I have experienced both extreme constipation – once I didn't go for 18 days in a row and the pain was awful – and I have also experienced frequent and very painful diarrhoea. I've also had a few horrible experiences where I haven't even been able to control my bowel, which ended in tears and upset.

IBS has impacted me emotionally, as it can be incredibly draining. Some of the more unrelenting symptoms can be scary. I would lay in bed every night worrying myself silly that something was seriously wrong. I don't enjoy going out at all because I'm always worried about needing to have a toilet nearby, but I can also feel too uncomfortable to even use a public toilet, and the thought of trying to eat and drink when I'm out and having to experience the bloating and pain. It's just all a bit much really, isn't it!

I have lost friends over the years because my IBS has had an impact on my social life. I find it very difficult staying at other people's houses, which people have found confusing and boring in the past. I also feel really nervous at the cinema when it's very quiet and my stomach starts making seriously questionable noises and people turn and stare. It's difficult to feel in control of the noises your body can make sometimes. Working out my trigger foods was a huge help in terms of managing my symptoms and I have to avoid wheat and gluten now, which has made a huge difference. I started a low FODmap diet which also helped a lot. Onions and garlic are my kryptonite. I minimise dairy and have a mug of hot water before meals and then a peppermint tea afterwards. I eat small portions more regularly throughout the day and this has helped.

I have always felt embarrassed about telling other people my issues and at school, I remember I used to wait until my lessons had started so that I could use the toilets when they were empty. Luckily, my boyfriend is so supportive and I feel so comfortable going to his house and sharing my worries with him. He is so patient and caring and understanding. It can be exhausting to hide your IBS symptoms and I think it's so important to communicate with your loved ones about what you are going through, as it takes such a weight off. Don't ignore your symptoms and find a healthcare professional who you feel comfortable with. Don't be afraid to ask for a second opinion and share your worries, concerns and symptoms with the people around you. Find your comforts and communicate. Don't keep it all bottled up inside."

"My gut health started to decline whilst I was in my first year of university. I was very stressed and unhappy – I think that's where it all began. The foods that I was told to stop eating by my doctor, as a result of my diagnosis, was the hardest thing to take. It definitely changed my life somewhat. I remember being happy that I had a diagnosis but I soon came to realise that being diagnosed with IBS didn't really help anything, since there's no one direct 'cure'.

The typical symptoms I have are bloating, painful gas, cramps and backache. For most of my IBS life, I've struggled massively with chronic constipation which has recently started being a bit more mixed, from constipation to diarrhoea. Basically, nothing seems to function very well. I also struggle a lot with fatigue and I feel my mental health suffers as a result of my IBS. The effects on my mental health are horrible a lot of the time. I find that IBS really does have a never-ending cycle with mental health. You can be struggling badly with anxiety, for example, and that can bring on the more physical symptoms of IBS which then, in turn, can make you feel more anxious to go out, for example. It's been never-ending for me.

Soon after my IBS diagnosis, I started to struggle with disordered eating which then grew into a full-blown eating disorder, which I spent time in a unit for. My IBS didn't cause my eating disorder, but it didn't help it either (my eating disorder made my IBS worse too). I also find that even now, whilst I'm in eating disorder recovery, my IBS affects me big time. It's harder to recover when you are in constant pain whenever you eat something. It doesn't help your relationship with food very much. I've never been the most confident person anyway and am quite introverted, but all the symptoms that comes along with IBS (physically AND mentally) have made me a lot less sociable. I've never been one for having lots of friends and IBS certainly didn't help me to maintain friendships. I mean, I'm hardly going to go out when none of my clothes fit me due to bloating and I'm farting every couple of minutes.

I have tried a huge amount of medication alongside my GP, none of which I would say has been successful. I was placed on the low FODMAP diet by a registered dietician which has definitely helped the most. I discovered foods that were triggers for my symptoms, and by removing them, I have been able to reduce my symptoms a lot. However, I still struggle every single day. As my IBS stems from stress, I believe that changing my diet isn't going to ever be the only answer. When things are at their worst, nothing works better for me than a hot water bottle, peppermint tea and an early night. I struggled my way through university for a number of reasons but my IBS was definitely a factor. It affected my academic and social life. Equally, my career in digital marketing was very intense at times, and I found I couldn't cope with the pressure and stress it brought. What I do now – working for myself full time – is probably the best thing I could have done for my IBS. I can work at my own pace, from home, with my dog on my lap. It just works. I'm more productive and efficient than I have ever been.

I actually feel really fortunate that I met my boyfriend prior to IBS. We have been together about 10 years now so we are very comfortable around each other. He also has IBS which is actually a massive bonus as we can relate to each other big time. Intimacy-wise, it definitely has an effect. I mean I usually end up going to bed with an IBS attack, plenty of bloating and gas. It doesn't really help in terms of being intimate. When I go to bed, I often just want to curl up and sleep the pain off... not do anything else!! I don't just have one, but my most embarrassing symptom is farting, for sure. That's what I've always struggled with the most. In the early days of my relationship, I'd try to rush out of the room to fart anywhere that Mark wasn't. Being at the gym and squatting, I let a fart out that turns out to be smelly, and have to pretend it wasn't me. Attempting silent farts in uni exams (because exams = nerves = IBS attack) was a real art of mine. Oh, and the classic, just sitting in a public toilet waiting for someone to use the hand dryer so you can let rip. I mean... we've all been there, right?!

When it comes to IBS, make sure your doctor has checked you out for everything else first. Symptoms that could be

IBS related could also be something else more serious – be mindful and get it checked. I'd really recommend seeing a registered dietitian too. Never try any sort of diet without one to guide you through it. You need their support to do it correctly! Also, never let anyone put your IBS down. Just because there are more serious conditions out there doesn't mean that you shouldn't let them do it. It's #notjustIBS – IBS can affect us as humans in so many ways, it can be so debilitating. IBS needs to be spoken about even more.

We need to destroy that Poo Taboo. I mean, as someone who is mostly constipated, pooing is my favourite thing to do!"

"I was diagnosed with the IBS a little over four years ago after suffering years of cramping and other digestive symptoms which I tried to ignore. I was relieved to have a diagnosis but unsure of what to do with this new information and how it would affect me. My main symptoms are crippling stomach cramps, constipation, wind and occasional nausea.

Depending on dietary and emotional factors, my symptoms can affect me daily but mostly around 3-4 times a week. I have found that my condition affects me emotionally. It's confusing and often frustrating as people who don't suffer with it don't understand. I suppose it can be a little lonely which doesn't help with symptoms at all. I often find that my condition affects my social life, as I have had to cancel plans or leave early due to my IBS symptoms.

The best advice I can give is to make sure you explain to other parties about your condition and they should be understanding. Also, try and find ways to control your symptoms, such as amending your diet and trying to limit stress or other triggers in the lead up to any big events. Through trial and error, I'm still figuring out my triggers and trying to work out how to live my best life with my condition. IBS is a painful and often embarrassing condition which can be debilitating at times. There has been a number of occasions where I have had to leave classes or leave work early due to stomach cramping or poo problems. It's not ideal. I once had a terrible flare-up about 45 minutes before I was due to start work. I was still stuck on the loo 10 minutes before the start of my shift. I had to call my boss from the toilet and explain the situation I was in and that I was going to be late. Anyone who has IBS knows that a flare-up loo session isn't the most silent of activities. The advice I'd give to someone who has had a recent diagnosis would be to try your hardest to figure out your triggers – mine are gluten, dairy and high FODMAP foods – and eliminate them as best you can to reduce irritation and symptoms. Also, look at your personal life and try to remove variables that might cause you stress. It's easier said than done, but it really does help."

"I was diagnosed with IBS when I was almost 16. It was a big shock and called for a huge lifestyle change as prior to this I had never had to think in great depth about the foods I was eating and how they would affect my body.

I was frustrated more than anything that I couldn't just eat like a 'normal' person but now I am grateful as it's made me more mindful and aware of the nutritional benefits of food. Let's just say THE BLOAT IS REAL. As the day goes, things just get progressively worse and whenever my gut is unhappy I feel down. It's hard to push on and act like nothing is wrong when all you want to do is curl up in bed and sleep things off.

As someone who is also very passionate about fitness, it really bothers me when I feel like something I don't have a lot of control of can control things like my performance and motivation. This is something that gets to me quite a lot, as when I am having an IBS flare-up I tend to distance myself from my boyfriend and sleep in a separate room. I think explaining to your friends and loved ones how you are feeling will help as the last thing you want is to be made feel guilty for cancelling or being a bit down in the dumps – literally!

My IBS has definitely made me a stronger person as I have lost count of the amount of times I have just had to suck it up and go into work or school, even when I was feeling hideous. It never gets easier but knowing when to prioritise your health is important.

Find what works for YOU in terms of diet. There is a lot of information out on the internet which is great but no two people (or stomachs) are the same, so take things slow and it will get easier over time."

GRACE'S STORY

"My main issue in the beginning was a very bloated stomach, to the point I looked pregnant, despite me usually being a size 10-12. However, the more bothersome symptoms now include a swollen tummy, nausea and abdominal pain. Depending on how my symptoms are, I can either want to eat everything in sight or go off food completely. There's always a dull ache in my stomach that can also heighten to become sharp shooting and stabbing pains. It varies a lot and can be extremely painful. I do occasionally have to stop what I'm doing, breathe hard, close my eyes and wince, and then I can carry on.

I read so much online about how IBS can affect your sex life and to start with I just brushed it off and thought – not me! But sadly, it's true and at times, when my symptoms are flaring up, the thought of having sex just annoys me as I suddenly don't feel sexy at all. My partner is very understanding, despite me often feeling like I'm letting him down.

I get emotional about my symptoms a lot, in part because I'm frustrated and want answers. And also because I am in pain a lot of the time. The most frustrating thing is that other people can think you're using it as an excuse not to do something, or worse, they say, 'Oh, I'm so bloated too,' and they reiterate to me that everyone gets bloated and that it's normal. A little bloating here and there is normal, but the extent to which I bloat and how often it is, is underestimated. It would be debilitating for anyone as it's so difficult to monitor and so severe.

Sometimes I just want to snuggle at home with a hot water bottle and not dress up to go out, as I don't feel like it. The other thing I have to consider is my choice of outfit. I can't wear anything too tight because I need to allow space for my tummy when it swells. There's nothing more upsetting than going out in something form-fitting and looking pregnant. It can be very draining to have to always think about your IBS and consider how it might impact your day.

Initially, I felt as though I was letting people down, but now I realise that if they are real friends they will understand. Just never beat yourself up over it or feel guilty. I wouldn't say it's impacted my career but it is hard to go to the toilet when I work in an office because when I have to go, I HAVE to go. I have absolutely no control whatsoever so in a way, it has impacted that side of things because it can be so embarrassing!! Plus, no-one at work knows because I keep it quite private and just deal with each day as it comes, so it's so hard to keep smiling through all the pain so that my colleagues don't suspect anything!

Stay in touch with your doctor and keep them updated on any new symptoms, as sometimes symptoms can change, worsen and cause more problems than they did before. It's so important to visit them and reassure yourself that you're being checked out as much as you can."

FAYE'S STORY

"My main symptoms are bloating, diarrhoea and stomach cramps, which on a bad week, I can experience daily. I work in retail so this can be really difficult. I get a little anxious if I'm out and about and my stomach begins to talk to me, especially when there are limited toilets around. Even then, I don't want to go into a public toilet when there may be queues of people waiting for me to finish, which then gives me "poo fright" as I like to call it.

I have cancelled plans in the past due to a flare-up, but I try to carry on living my life as normal. Most of my friends and family know what my bowels are like so I visit their houses without worry or embarrassment, as they understand that I'll be spending a lot of time in their bathroom.

I'd advise being honest and open about your condition with your loved ones; it makes it easier for you to carry on living your life as normal without feeling unnecessary shame. It also helps to be open with your managers too. In fact, it has become a running joke in my workplace about how much I need to go to the bathroom.

I don't mind what my other half thinks of my bowels and he doesn't care either. I can be as intimate as I like with him, and I can tell him that I need to go ASAP. Just this weekend when we were in London, I had to use the bathroom and I was in there for a *while*. My boyfriend kept asking me if I was okay and I was like, "Yeah, just having a lot of poos." He laughed and that was that. I always complain to him about my tummy aches and my bad wind. He finds it funny which is great for me because I can just be myself around him and not put on some kind of act like I'm the "perfect woman", which I am definitely not.

Try not to let your symptoms affect your life more than they should. Be sure to still go out and have fun, but I would advise always scouting for the nearest loo beforehand because you never know when you're going to need one. And information is power, as they say!"

"I discovered I had IBS at the age of 35, after having horrible stomach cramps, diarrhoea, constipation and pain. It seemed to get worse around my periods. I was devastated, and at the same time, relieved that someone had a "name" for what I was going through.

Since going gluten and dairy free about five years ago, I only have the occasional flare-up caused by anxiety. Travel can be a nightmare, especially long car trips or excursions where I worry about whether there will be a bathroom. I bring my own food when available, but that isn't always possible, especially on a vacation. So I tend to I plan ahead and I bring a cooler of food and book a hotel with a kitchenette. If I am taking a cruise, I alert the cruise line ahead of time.

I always have to consider invitations. I sometimes decline because I know that there will be no gluten-free options. I am tired of saying, "I can't". It took me 15 years to realise that gluten and dairy were making my condition worse. A lot of lost work days and some lost jobs because of excessive absence. I was a customer service rep for many years and being on the phone when you have to "go" is an issue. Also, being away from your desk for extended periods.

Having IBS actually brought my husband and I closer together. I met my husband on Match.com just before I was diagnosed with gallbladder disease. He had only known me around a couple of months, but he took care of me after gallbladder surgery. He has gracefully dealt with my "tummy issues" for twenty years. So I knew he was a "keeper" from very early on. My advice to anyone suffering from digestive symptoms is to get tested for coeliac disease. Try eliminating gluten, and then dairy to see if that helps too."

"My main IBS symptoms seem to be pain, wind and bloating, which affect me most days. The emotional symptoms of IBS are definitely the most difficult to deal with. I think the anxiety and depression related to IBS mainly come from the fact that you can feel low in self-confidence as the symptoms can be quite isolating. They can leave you stuck in your own thoughts, which can be unkind to yourself.

I've found that IBS has shaken my confidence quite a bit, it has made me conscious of what I'm wearing due to bloating and pain. A lot of the time I don't feel like 'me' anymore due to not wearing the items of clothing I actually WANT to wear. I find that when I'm feeling anxious, my symptoms worsen and I can barely move away from the bathroom, whilst when I'm feeling depressed, I don't manage my diet well, as I just want to eat comfort foods which can trigger my IBS.

IBS has certainly had an impact on my social life! I once loved going out with friends, especially for food, but I now feel unable to. As soon as I eat my symptoms begin and it is really hard to concentrate on socialising when you're in so much pain. Unfortunately, I've had a few 'friends' who weren't understanding about it, and it's really hard when you lose friends over something that you can't control. My advice would be to ignore those who don't understand, they aren't real friends anyway! Also, try and make plans with friends which won't be affected by your symptoms, such as a girl's night in.

I have had my diagnosis for nearly a year now, and I still haven't completely found a management plan that works for me. I haven't yet found specific trigger foods as I have tried cutting out a lot of different foods at different times. So currently, I feel like food in general sets my IBS off! I was also given medication alongside my diagnosis which didn't work, so I'm still trying to figure out a management plan.

Luckily, IBS has never had an impact on my relationship. My boyfriend and I were friends before we were together so we have always been quite open with each other, and one of his siblings suffers from IBD so he understands stomach issues very well! However, from my side of the relationship, I do feel very unsexy with my bloated stomach and it can get me down sometimes.

Obviously, at the beginning of a relationship, you don't fart around each other and with IBS it can be quite hard to hold them in. At the beginning of our relationship, I'd been holding one in for quite a while one evening and my boyfriend made me laugh. Unfortunately for me, it slipped out, which he found absolutely hilarious. I went bright red and covered my face for what felt like an eternity. He still mentions it now because he still finds it funny. I'm so glad that he wasn't disgusted as I couldn't help it!

Don't panic, you are not alone and there are a lot of people to talk to about IBS, as well as the IBS Network. More people suffer from the condition than you think and we're all very open about it! It is manageable once you've found your management plan!

If you're struggling to get a diagnosis, persevere with going to the GP. IBS is a lot easier to understand and manage once you've received your diagnosis."

"I discovered I was suffering from IBS when I visited the doctors with tummy pain and a severe food intolerance. At first, I was relieved to find out what was wrong, but at the same time, I was upset as IBS isn't a 'pinpointed' issue. I suffer most with food intolerance, bloating, cramping, changes in bowel movements, fatigue and anxiety. It's always been something I've been embarrassed about as no-one talks openly about it, yet a large percentage of the population suffers with it!

I'm a lot better at coping with my symptoms now as I have a clearer view on my 'trigger' foods, but in the beginning, I found it really embarrassing and upsetting as I'd have to miss out on opportunities because I would have to say at home in bed, in agony!

The amount of events and plans with friends that I've had to cancel because of a flare-up is staggering! If you know you have somewhere to go or a social event, I would suggest you eat plain foods the day before and make sure that you look at what you're eating while you're out.

At home, it's not as embarrassing. You're in your own home, so you can rest and make a hot water bottle. When you are out, it can send your anxiety sky high! I know it varies from person to person, but it took me a good year to find a diet that I was comfortable with after identifying my trigger foods. Symptoms can be extremely inconvenient too. A few years ago, I booked Disneyland for my birthday and unfortunately had a high flare-up, so I couldn't enjoy it or go on any rides. It was my 18th birthday and supposed to be a special one, but I suppose it's an excuse to book another trip! I found that changing my diet and eliminating foods which I knew would set my IBS off helped no end! Also, a big one (for me) was reducing stress levels. Stress can trigger IBS, as emotion hits your gut first. So it's always best to look into ways of reducing your stress levels whenever possible."

"My first experience with IBS coincided with the start of my new job, which was based in Central London and involved me getting the tube into work every day. The most problematic symptom for me was diarrhoea, which would invariably strike as I was making my way to my office. I had some really horrible experiences, including one memorable occasion where a train was stuck at a red signal for what seemed like an eternity and my stomach audibly cried out for the toilet. It was mortifying.

I think initially, IBS can be a complete minefield because the symptoms are so alien and so brand new. However as you learn to accept and get used to your body, it becomes less scary - because you can anticipate certain symptoms and manage them accordingly. Scarlett actually encouraged me to speak to my boss, which helped immensely as he accommodated my suggestion of flexible working - which meant that I could come into work a little later (and miss the peak train rush) or work from home, depending on the severity of my symptoms on any given day.

Don't be afraid to speak out - and talk to other sufferers. You can feel so alone in the beginning and often, this isolation can heighten your symptoms. Don't let IBS take control, you've got this!"

I TRULY DO BELIEVE THAT THE KEY TO

UNLOCKING THE 'STIGMA' ASSOCIATED

WITH THE 'POO TABOO' IS TO KEEP AN

OPEN, HONEST AND FRANK DIALOGUE

ABOUT IBS GOING. THERE IS NO SHAME,

NO EMBARRASSMENT AND NO NEED

TO FEEL ALONE.

I don't know about you but the idea of changing my diet was pretty overwhelming initially.

Cheese, chocolate and ice cream were staple parts of my diet, so I wasn't quite certain how I'd be able to overhaul it completely.

But having lost control of my body to the symptoms of IBS, I was determined to try out a new way of eating to see if I could alleviate my issues.

CHAPTER 12

Recipes &
Food Plan Ideas

I wouldn't necessarily advise everyone to go completely cold turkey like I did, but I'm pretty 'all or nothing' when it comes to food. I've spent years wishing I was one of those disciplined people who could have just ONE square of chocolate before returning the bar to the fridge and saving it for the following day.

But I'm not.

I eat the ENTIRE packet of biscuits. OR I put them into the bin.

And so that's exactly what I did with my kitchen cupboards when I finally made the decision to overhaul my eating to a far more 'tummy friendly' plan.

I swiped the cupboards of biscuits, chocolate, cereals, cakes, cereal bars, long-life milk, packet sauces and gravies. I cleared the fridge of cheese, butter, milk and cream, and donated anything unopened to a food bank.

And I started from scratch.

I did a lot of online research and put together a very basic but nutritious meal plan of fail-safe tummy soothing recipes.

I started off pretty basic (i.e. very little in the way of flavourings, herbs, spices etc. for fear of setting off a trigger) and then slowly reintroduced more 'adventurous' concoctions.

Once again, I must reiterate, I am not a nutritionist, help expert, dietician or doctor. These are just some very simple tummy-friendly, soothing recipes to provide inspiration if you're struggling to find things to eat.

Obviously, it is just a guideline because you might have a far smaller appetite than I do. I quite literally eat for England and have a BIG meal for breakfast, lunch and dinner. But you can tweak these depending on how hungry you are. Remember the motto – eat to make your body happy. Listen to your body and use what you put into it as a way of becoming more in tune with how it reacts. I found, initially, that eating little and often was most effective, before being able to tweak it accordingly and then gradually increased the size of my meals.

EXAMPLE WEEKLY FOOD PLAN
(recipes below):

MONDAY
Breakfast: almond milk porridge with fruit

Lunch: leftover roast

Dinner: chicken fajitas and guacamole

Snack: carrot sticks and hummus

TUESDAY
Breakfast: almond milk porridge with berries

Lunch: leftover chicken fajitas and guacamole

Dinner: jacket potato with tuna

Snack: rice cakes and almond butter

WEDNESDAY
Breakfast: banana oat pancakes with coconut yoghurt

Lunch: chicken salad wrap

Dinner: chicken, vegetables and rice

Snack: mashed avocado on Ryvita

THURSDAY

Breakfast: bran flakes with plain soya yoghurt

Lunch: chicken, vegetables and rice

Dinner: Pasta Scarbonara

Snack: carrot sticks and hummus

FRIDAY

Breakfast: homemade granola with coconut yoghurt

Lunch: wrap pizza

Dinner: salmon, sweet potato, avocado & strawberry salad

Snack: rice cake and aubergine dip (baba ganoush)

SATURDAY

Breakfast: homemade granola with coconut yoghurt

Lunch: Pasta Scarbonara

Dinner: creamy vegetable risotto

Snack: oatcakes, topped with almond butter and banana slices

SUNDAY

Breakfast: banana oat pancakes with maple syrup

Lunch: chicken salad

Dinner: Sunday tummy friendly 'roast'

Snack: watermelon pieces

BREAKFAST OPTIONS

I go through phases of having the same breakfast day in, day out, until I'm totally sick of it. I tend to find my body really likes routine and getting the same amount of fibre first thing in the morning, without fail. My breakfast is a 'signal' to my body to go to the toilet, and I have somewhat trained my body to do this, so that I can get the toilet trip out of the way before I leave the house for the day. I tend to have a large mug of peppermint tea with my breakfast every morning which helps to wake my body up – and ignite the bowels. And I also find drinking a large glass of water in the mornings can also provide much-needed assistance. This is my 'fail-safe' formula. And it's pretty effective.

Porridge

Porridge is a quick, easy and cheap breakfast that fills you up. It keeps you warm during those frosty winter mornings and is packed with plenty of soluble fibre, which keeps your insides healthy and ensures you stay regular. It's an ideal breakfast if you suffer from IBS-C and are unsure of where to start. In the US, it's referred to as 'oatmeal', but it's essentially the same concept – one cup of porridge oats (I prefer Scottish oats, but they all do the trick), to one cup water (or plant-based milk), then you pop in the microwave for two minutes. Eventually, you find the consistency you like most (I prefer mine a little watery) so you can add more or less liquid, but it's so soothing on your tummy and such a staple in my diet. Sweeten with maple syrup or berries. While you are figuring out triggers, it may be best to avoid artificial sweeteners, only because they can sometimes bloat you or give you a laxative effect. I had a very unfortunate experience recently when I ate an entire tub of vegan ice cream, not realising it was full of sweetener. I spent the rest of the evening farting and the following morning on the toilet.

Homemade granola

One of my all-time favourite breakfasts is my homemade granola, which takes a little bit of extra preparation but it's oh so worth it, I can assure you. You'll need a big airtight jar to store your granola in once it's cooked, but it means you can make up several weeks' worth in one batch and it's such a quick, easy and delicious breakfast option. You'll need a big bag of giant oats, sunflower seeds, cacao powder, dried white mulberries (or a dried berry of your choice, I just prefer them), coconut oil, coconut sugar and almond milk. Blend the cacao powder, sunflower seeds, mulberries, coconut sugar and 2 tbsp's of almond milk in a blender. It doesn't need to be completely smooth, but you want it to have a slightly wet consistency. Line a baking tray and put a tbsp of coconut oil on it, before popping it in an oven at 180 degrees. Pour the giant oats into a mixing bowl and then pour in the cacao/seeds/sugar mix. Stir the mixture until the oats are coated in the mix. Take the baking tray out of the oven after 3-4 minutes (the coconut oil should be melted) and pour your oats mix onto the tray. Drizzle some maple syrup on top of the mix. Bake for approximately 25-35 minutes until golden brown and leave to cool before decanting into your airtight container. Have a scoop of your granola every morning with a dollop of plain coconut yoghurt. Delicious!

Banana oat pancakes

This is definitely something to have when you have a little bit more time on your hands, so it's a great weekend breakfast option! The riper the banana is, the better this seems to taste too! Mash up one small banana into a mixing bowl, then add approximately one cup oats and a slosh of almond milk (depends on the size of your banana and oats but, generally, the consistency shouldn't be too wet – just sticky enough to stick together). Then you can get creative with what you'd like your pancakes to feature – blueberries, cacao powder (if you'd like a bit of a chocolate fix), cacao nibs. Heat a small dollop of coconut oil in a pan and add the mix to the pan in small portions (I usually make three small pancakes). Fry on a low heat, flipping after 5-10 minutes until each side is golden brown. Serve with maple syrup, berries or a sprinkling of sugar.

LUNCH OPTIONS

Pasta Scarbonara

As I'm sure you may have deduced already, before my IBS troubles surfaced, I was ever so slightly invested in my love for cheese. Cheesy pasta was a university staple and while I definitely DO NOT miss the bloated, gassy feeling after consuming a generous bowl of it, I do miss the comfort of a big bowl of pasta. I initially found a number of recipes involving cashews and butternut squash as a creamy 'cheese replacement'; however, unfortunately, cashews make my throat swell up (I'm a bundle of laughs, aren't I?), so it was back to the drawing board.

I tried not to use the supermarket cheese replacements as they were full of quite a lot of ingredients that I didn't quite recognise, so eventually I came up with a rather basic recipe of my very own. You can certainly get more adventurous with it as time goes on but it's a good place to start.

Introducing pasta 'Scarbonara' (as in a 'Scar'lett special; honestly, my creative talents are wasted aren't they…). To enjoy this fine dish, you'll need a packet of nutritional yeast, which is super high in B12. I usually purchase it from a health food shop. It smells and looks a little bit like what I used to feed my fish. But I promise looks are deceiving, it can be used as a cheese replacement for a variety of dishes and it's a great staple for your cupboards. You'll also need a chicken or vegetable stock cube, some unsweetened almond milk, a pinch of black pepper and a dried pasta of your choice. OR if you want to make it healthier and more fibrous then you could try some 'konjac flour noodles'. These are often sold as 'zero calorie/carb noodles or pasta' and, again, can be found in health food stores, but I love them not for their low-calorie benefits but because they are very high in fibre. Cook the pasta in one pan (the konjac noodles only tend to need 4-5 minutes on the boil) and heat the almond milk (one cup) in another with the stock cube for around 5 minutes on a medium heat. Then slowly add in sprinklings of nutritional yeast until the consistency thickens up to resemble more of a sauce. You'll usually find you'll need quite a fair amount of nutritional yeast, so don't be afraid to keep adding it in. Pop in the pasta and ta-dah! You can add other ingredients, such as smoked salmon, sweetcorn, peas, spinach, chopped sage, parsley etc. too! Customise your pasta to your hearts content.

Wrap Pizza

Do you sense a theme here? I've definitely tried to make some of my favourite meals into tummy-friendly, healthier versions and over the years, although I've had some real disasters, I do seem to have found some really simple ideas that allow me to have 'pizza' and 'pasta' while not irritating my sensitive stomach. For the wrap pizza, all you need is wholemeal or white tortilla wraps, tomato puree, vegetables and nutritional yeast. Pre-heat the oven on a low-medium heat, put the wrap on a baking tray with a teeny bit of olive oil, spread over the tomato puree, load up your veggies (I love sweetcorn, spinach and broccoli, but it's totally up to you) and sprinkle on the nutritional yeast for a cheesy hit. Stick it in the oven for 8-10 minutes and out comes – pizza!

DINNER OPTIONS

Chicken Fajitas & Guacamole

Chicken Fajitas are a staple part of my diet, largely because they are so quick, easy and simple to make, but they also really seem to love my tummy. Thankfully! Avocado is a really great food if you have IBS-C because it's full of fibre and good fats to help get things moving and grooving in your intestines!

Usually, chicken fajitas are made with peppers and onions. However, some people are a little sensitive to night-shades (that's peppers and tomatoes to you and me) and onions, so I switch things up and pop in small chunks of butternut squash, baby corn, carrot, courgette and any other veg that you find a 'safe bet'. Sprinkle on a fajita mix (or create your own, it's usually made up of paprika, cayenne pepper and cumin), mash up some avocado with some salt, fry it up and pop it into a tortilla wrap. Usually, there's quite a lot of mix here, so I'll pack up a spare wrap in some tinfoil for lunch the next day.

Salmon, sweet potato & strawberry salad

Now, I can't quite take credit for the strawberry salad because it's the special recipe of my friends Misha and Kasha, but this amazing dinner is one of my favourites and it seems to love my tummy too. Bake the salmon in the oven with a drizzle of oil, wrapped in tinfoil and with a dusting of salt and pepper (30-35 minutes). Also, bake the sweet potato in the oven too (it just doesn't quite taste the same when it's been in the microwave). Another secret tip from Misha is to drizzle some maple syrup onto the sweet potato. It adds an amazing sweetness to the skin, which is the most fibre-filled part and definitely too delicious to miss. For the strawberry salad mix ripe avocado pieces, strawberry pieces, leaves, pomegranate seeds and cucumber slices. Delicious!

Sunday Tummy Friendly Roast

A roast dinner has always been a staple in our household; however, I always used to find that it would upset my stomach and leave me ending the week on a sour note (i.e. sat on the toilet). It wasn't until quite recently that I realised this was because most supermarket gravy granules have milk powder in them. Marvellous. So I now make a slightly downsized version, so as not to overload my stomach with food all in one go. I'll do a big roast chicken, roast potatoes (sliced small, cooked in an oil of your choice – I tend to use olive oil and sprinkled with rosemary), maple glazed roasted carrots, peas, sweetcorn and vegetable 'free from' gravy. Just be sure to check what's in the ingredients. The only thing I've noticed is that my stomach seems to be fine with the roast on the day, but once the potatoes have cooled in the fridge and then been reheated, the starch created by this process can make my tummy a little gassy. So it's best to eat all the potatoes on the day and then save the chicken and veg leftovers for the week! Any excuse for extra potatoes, eh?

Sesame tomato chicken, quinoa and roasted veg

Okay, so it sounds a bit boring – but it's actually really delicious. Fry off some chicken with a teaspoon of olive oil and slowly add in some plain tomato passata, basil, pepper, sage and Himalayan pink salt. You can add onion and garlic if you can tolerate it but I try and avoid it if I can. When the sauce is ready, sprinkle over a generous helping of sesame seeds (I can't get enough of these) and leave it to cool. Roast veg wise, I use sweet potato, courgette, red peppers and asparagus – topped with fresh rosemary and thyme – popped in a hot oven for 20 mins. Cook the quinoa plain or with the leftover tomato passata – to be enjoyed with your sesame chicken sauce! You can make up big batches of this to take into work/school for lunch.

DESSERTS

Melt in the middle chocolate mug cake and coconut cream

If you're really craving something sweet or need a replacement 'chocolate fix', then my go-to is a little invention which I now consider better than the family-size pack of Galaxy I used to consume on a daily basis (yes, honestly). Get yourself a mug and pop in one tablespoon of cacao powder (be sparing with this stuff, it's quite bitter – I'd pop in loads at first and wonder why it was so disgusting. It might be the raw form of chocolate but it's not the same – sorry!), 2 tablespoons of buckwheat flour (contrary to the name, it's wheat/gluten-free), about 75ml of rice milk and 2 tablespoons of pure maple syrup or honey (more if you want it sweeter). Stick it in the microwave for about 1 minute and while it's cooking away, dollop a spoonful of CoYo Vanilla Bean Yoghurt into a bowl. It's essentially coconut yoghurt but it's not overwhelmingly coconutty because of the vanilla. It honestly tastes like cream and it's amazing once you've scooped out your steaming melt-in-the-middle mug cake into the bowl too. Now I will warn you, this isn't the most picturesque of desserts. But it's absolutely delicious.

The overriding factor with your food plan should be about balance. The worst thing that you can do is to make yourself scared of food. It's more about striking up a healthy relationship so that you are very in tune with how each thing you put into your body reacts with your symptoms.

I personally don't have any experience of disordered eating, but I do appreciate how dangerous it can be to get yourself into a cycle of being afraid of how food will exacerbate your symptoms. There was a time in my final year of university where I found myself limiting things a little TOO much and so I had to really look closely at my relationship with food and scale back on how restrictive I was being.

Remember to always consult a nutritionist or GP whenever entering into any kind of elimination diet.

As a handy checklist to keep on you (because I do hope this will be a guide you keep coming back to), I've included below my go-to list of tummy friendly foods. Many are high in fibre (both the soluble and insoluble kind) and should definitely be woven into our day-to-day eating pattern wherever possible. They are all foods that I'm able to eat with no problems at all, but obviously, everyone is different!

Stock up on:

- O STRAWBERRIES

- O AVOCADO

- O BANANAS

- O CARROTS

- O LENTILS

- O BROCCOLI

- O BEETROOT

- O ARTICHOKE

- O QUINOA

- O OATS

- O CHIA SEEDS

- O SWEET POTATO

- O RAW CACAO POWDER

- O KIWI

- O WATERMELON

- O CHICKEN

- O SALMON

- O COD

- O FLAT FISH

- TROUT

- PARSNIPS

- BUTTERNUT SQUASH

- COURGETTE

- SPINACH

- LETTUCE

- KALE

- BLUEBERRIES

- OLIVES

- NUTS

- SEEDS

- COCONUT YOGHURT

- RICE

- RICE, OAT, ALMOND OR COCONUT MILK

- MAPLE SYRUP

- RICE CAKES

- POTATOES

- DATES

ALTERNATIVE TREATS

Just because you're sticking to an IBS friendly plan, doesn't mean that you can't enjoy a few treats from time to time. Cutting out dairy definitely eliminated a lot of traditionally high-sugar and calorific treats, such as chocolate, cake, cheese and ice cream, which helped me to have a healthier balance of what I put into my body.

In the beginning, I tried not to buy any dairy-free 'alternatives' because many of them seemed to feature a lot of ingredients I didn't recognise (which was my buffer in the initial stages of transforming my eating pattern). However, I now like to enjoy them as part of a balanced diet. Here are some of my favourites! I often whip these out at any dinner parties we are hosting and no-one has ever complained. In fact, I may have even converted a few seasoned chocoholics!

BOOJA BOOJA - a creamy, decadent ice cream made from just water, cashew nuts, cocoa powder and syrup. They also do amazing chocolate truffles – the salted caramel is my favourite!

MOO FREE - they offer a delicious range of dairy-free chocolate

VIOLIFE CHEESE - the cheese slices are my favourites, perfect for adding a cheesy topping to fajitas or pizza

SWEDISH GLACE - delicious vanilla pod ice cream

ALMOND DREAM - salted caramel ice cream - yum!

ALPRO – they offer dairy-free custards, yoghurts, desserts and ice creams, all with a soya base

BEN & JERRY'S DAIRY FREE - use their web checker to see which stores near you stock the DF version

COCOA LIBRE - another of my favourite dairy-free chocolate brands, made with rice milk for the ultimate creamy chocolatey taste! They also do chocolate reindeers and Santa's at Christmas time, if you want to inform any relatives that you don't have to miss out on sweet gifts!

LIVIA'S KITCHEN - made with natural ingredients such as dates, oat flour, maple syrup etc. You can often find her delicious treats in high street stores and they are perfect for on-the-go treats. If you were also a Millionaire's Shortbread addict prior to going dairy-free (I once ate an entire family Millionaire's Cheesecake in one sitting; I say once, it may have happened several times) then give the raw millionaire bites a try! You may just be converted, forever!

OMBAR CHOCOLATE - another favourite of mine for decadent, luxuriously creamy chocolate (definitely helping satiate any Galaxy bar cravings I used to have), the Coco

Mylk bar is the chocolate of dreams and the Coco Mylk chocolate buttons are incredible.

Oreos and Biscoff biscuits are 'accidentally' dairy-free too, as they contain soya instead of any milk products.

Some of the Candy Kittens sweet flavours are gelatine and dairy-free, and come in snack packs for a more reserved treat (rather than the giant bags, which I can't help but devour).

Obviously, everything in moderation, but make sure you enjoy and love your food and learn to discover the foods that love you back!

I WISH I COULD DEVELOP THE MAGIC

FORMULA FOR A CURE AND SEND YOU

ALL A BIG BOTTLE, BUT AS I'M SURE YOU'LL

HAVE GATHERED BY NOW, THAT'S NOT

WHAT IBS IS ABOUT.

Round-Up

So there, we have it. You now know my IBS life story and everything in between.

I hope that, if anything at all, you have laughed at some of my perils and realised you're definitely not alone in your IBS struggles.

There's no overnight fix or quick solution, which makes the condition even more frustrating to deal with.

I wish I could develop the magic formula for a cure and send you all a big bottle, but as I'm sure you'll have gathered by now, that's not what IBS is about.

However, there are many things you can try to regain control of your body, minimise the impact your symptoms are having on your daily life and ensure you aren't suffering in silence. We've covered each of these topics in more detail in other chapters of the book, but here's a quick round-up:

- IDENTIFY WHICH TYPE OF IBS YOU SUFFER FROM AND WHAT YOUR MAIN SYMPTOMS ARE.

- DO AS MUCH RESEARCH AS YOU CAN ON IBS AND START TO BUILD UP A LIST OF THINGS YOU MIGHT LIKE TO TRY OR CONSULT YOUR GP ABOUT

- VISIT YOUR DOCTOR TO RULE OUT OTHER CONDITIONS AND UNDERGO TESTS

- KEEP A FOOD DIARY TO IDENTIFY YOUR TRIGGER FOODS AND BECOME MORE IN TUNE WITH YOUR BODY

- VISIT A NUTRITIONIST TO SEE WHAT EATING PLAN MIGHT WORK BEST FOR YOU

- WEAVE SOME GENTLE EXERCISE INTO YOUR DAY

- CONFIDE IN SOMEONE. IT HELPS TO HAVE AN IBS ALLY YOU CAN GO TO TO AIR YOUR CONCERNS (IF YOU DON'T HAVE ONE, EMAIL ME!)

- MAKE SMALL, HELPFUL CHANGES TO YOUR DIET TO SEE WHAT IMPACT IT HAS ON YOUR IBS

- MAKE PLANS AT YOUR PLACE OF WORK OR SCHOOL TO ENSURE THAT YOU ARE GOING TO BE UNDERSTOOD AND BE ABLE TO MANAGE YOUR IBS ON A DAY-TO-DAY BASIS COMFORTABLY.

- EXERCISE SELF-LOVE AND KINDNESS – TRY NOT TO PUNISH YOURSELF WHEN YOUR IBS FLARES UP

O   LEARN TO LAUGH AND HAVE A SENSE OF HUMOUR.
    A POSITIVE MENTAL ATTITUDE CAN REALLY HELP
    WHEN APPROACHING FLARE-UPS

In the most simple form, I like to think of your IBS recovery starting as a three-prong approach:

O   MENTAL WELLBEING

O   FOOD

O   SUPPLEMENTS

In the mental wellbeing stage, you need to find a therapy or therapist that you can trust, confide in and figure out a way of dealing with all of the emotional complexities that IBS throws up. Whether this is CBT, hypnotherapy, mindfulness, coaching or counselling. Anxiety was a HUGE trigger for me and finding out ways to escape that catch 22 cycle was invaluable in getting to the bottom of my IBS.

Food is another overwhelming factor and trigger for IBS which has to be managed as effectively as possible in order to maximise your chances of a successful recovery. You shouldn't be scared of food, but look at it instead as a way of maturing your taste-buds, resetting the rut that we all get into with food and getting adventurous. When you highlight your trigger foods, you regain a huge sense of control over your symptoms and can minimise their impact.

And then, of course, supplements (and/or medication, depending on what's right for you) is the final step in creating that harmony within your body and setting the perfect grounds for a symptom-free life. Figuring out which supplements might be able to assist specific symptoms can be a lengthy process, but once you get there, you'll be so glad you persevered.

The food and therapy are the foundations and then the supplements can be a harmoniser.

It's a healing process that gets better with experience and time, but you WILL get there.

During the period of my life when I saw the MOST improvement in my symptoms, I realised that I had to REALLY want to get better. I know that might sound silly, as none of us wants to be poorly and ill all the time, but I had just accepted defeat so long and got myself into a seemingly inescapable dark cycle. I didn't WANT to get better because I didn't think it was possible. I wasn't ready to take back control because I pitied my situation and couldn't see an end to my symptoms on the horizon.

In the end, I had to face up to the fact that getting better wasn't going to happen overnight and wouldn't happen if I didn't make more permanent lifestyle changes. For so long, I'd be waiting for the magic pill to swoop in and take all my symptoms away without stopping to consider that there wasn't ever going to be one. In fact, the 'magic pill' was me making a pact with myself to kick-start my healthier, 'tummy friendly' habits, work on my mental wellbeing and investigate which supplements might boost the elements I was lacking.

I'm pleased to say that I now no longer consider IBS to be a disturbance in my life. It's no longer that hideous weight that I have to bear on my shoulders and hide from the world. I've accepted that it's one of my quirks. I've done tonnes of research, I've learned to laugh more, I've found the people who love me no matter what and I've found a career set up that works for me.

I still have bad days (or weeks) and good weeks, but I'd say I'm 95% better than how I was several years ago. I live an active, varied lifestyle and am symptom-free for the majority. Often, I can immediately pinpoint any flare-ups to external stressors (such as a work deadline) or accidental dairy consumption. But it's a reminder to bring myself back on track, and I actually sometimes NEED those reminders.

We can be so stuck in the rat race of life that we take things for granted. So I sometimes think my IBS pops back up to say hello as a reminder to slow down, be grateful for the wonderful people and opportunities I have in my life, enjoy myself, and live life to the full.

At the very end of this book, I've provided some 'next step' resources for you to look into. I can highly recommend each book personally and I implore you to do lots of research about IBS as a means of really figuring out what makes your body tick and how, ultimately, you can rid your body of the troublesome symptoms.

I wanted to find a way to round this book off positively, and since there's no 'well there we have it, you're cured' ending, I thought the best way to finish things on a productive note would be to leave you with the 9 rules that I live by.

They're not all IBS specific or even related to IBS symptoms in any way, but I'm sure if you look closely, you'll be able to see certain links to IBS and how I came to create the rules in the first place.

If you're already a reader of my blog (SCARLETTLONDON. COM), then you'll have probably already seen these rules. But here they are again, for good measure.

The 9 Rules I Live By

Life doesn't come with a rule book, which is both exciting and frustrating. Your life is yours to carve, yours to enjoy and yours to create memories.

But it can be tricky when there's a stumbling block because more often than not, we have to experience something in order to recognise how to deal with it.

Think of the first time you got a bad mark in school or fell out with a friend. This felt like the worst thing in the world because your experiences of going through it were limited.

Think about when you lost your first pet, it is your first experience of grief and of loss.

It's difficult to deal with, and while guidance from your parents can certainly help, you have to pull through and steer yourself in the right direction.

We learn something new every day, which is what makes life so varied and so interesting.

But in my *(almost)* 24 years of living, I have a set of small, flexible rules that I live by that keep my anxious thoughts at bay and help reassure me that I'm carving my path my own way.

I try not to compare it to the paths of others, but I allow myself to admire what those around me have created.

We're all following our own individual journey – and we all have our own stories to tell.

But while I'm still in the process of writing my story, here are just a few little rules that I think are important to recognise in everyday life.

1. Everyone is equal

You know when you get that anxious feeling when you're meeting someone important?

Or someone famous – or perhaps even a YouTuber you have watched for years?

It's anticipation that you have to be on your best behaviour, anticipation for what they'll be like and what they'll think of you.

Or perhaps you're meeting someone who is very wealthy or has an incredible job. Maybe they have an overwhelming number of followers on social media. You feel like you have to treat them in a certain way and you don't want to get it wrong. You don't want to step up and say the wrong thing. You feel like you have something to prove.

But really, we're all human.

We're all equals and regardless of what each individual chooses to do with their life, we're still all made of the same flesh and bone.

We all have to eat to survive and go to the toilet.

We all have problems (relative to our life) that fluctuate our mood and we all have a variety of experiences which shape us.

Very early on in our relationship, my boyfriend David taught me a vital life lesson – not to be intimidated by who you're meeting because, in the grand scheme of things, we are all equal. Don't put anyone on a pedestal because it doesn't gain anything. Admire but still appreciate their humanness. Just because somebody is richer, poorer, prettier, more glamorous, more successful or less qualified, everybody deserves to be treated with the same respect that you'd like others to show to you.

When you level everyone out onto an equal playing field, you can just be you, so let your best qualities shine, rather than let your nerves take over.

What happens next is what's supposed to be. *Which leads us onto the next life lesson...*

2. Not everyone will like you

I *reaaallly* struggled with this one for a long time because I'd always followed the mantra, treat others how you'd like to be treated, and so when somebody hurt my feelings, isolated me or was unkind, I thought it was a reflection of something I'd done.

I couldn't fathom why someone would be so cruel or criticise me unfairly when I hadn't mistreated them.

One book that really helped me overcome this confusion was *The Chimp Paradox*, which is a fabulous mind management model that helps you understand that we're not all perfect and sometimes we let our inner 'chimp' (or our inner child) take over.

We act irrationally.

We act in a way that has been shaped by our past experiences.

We have off days.

But more relevantly to this life lesson, not everyone will like us and we have to accept that in order to live happily.

It outlines that on average, out of five chimps, three will like you instantly, one could be swayed to like you with experience and one will never like you, regardless of how nice you are to them, how you treat them or how hard you try to win them over.

As the saying goes, you could be the juiciest peach in the basket but there will always be someone that doesn't like peaches.

Don't let someone else's opinion of you change your opinion of yourself.

Don't waste your finite time and energy trying to win over people that can't see your value.

It doesn't mean they are a bad person (or that you are), it just means they're not your cup of tea and you're not theirs.

That's okay.

Accept, move on, be polite but remember that you can't control what others think about you.

Be you, *the rest will fall into place.*

3. Eat to make your body and mind happy

This is a BIG one for me because I punished my body for so long on various different diets in a bid to lose weight.

I deprived myself of things, I counted calories, I didn't eat enough food.

I wasn't showing my body and mind the love it deserved. I wasn't providing it with the good fuel it needed.

I had totally the wrong mindset and I was fixated on aesthetics which blinded me from what really mattered.

Our bodies are amazing things, they come in all shapes and sizes.

They are hard-working machines which exude beauty, and we have the ultimate control of maintaining them and treating them well. You have to make your body happy.

And when I changed my mindset from, 'I want to look good and lose weight' to 'I want to make sure my body is happy and functioning properly,' it was like the dark cloud had lifted.

I didn't have to feel guilty anymore.

Admittedly, a lot of my initial motivation was sparked by the fact I was really poorly.

Aged 21, I was pretty much bed and bathroom bound with my troublesome tummy and I was fed up of it ruling my life.

I realised what I could control was making sure that I put food into my body which made it happy.

So, instead of eating a huge gooey chocolate cake (which admittedly satiated my cravings in the moment, as it can give the impression it's making your body 'happy') and feeling tired, sluggish, sick and bloated afterwards, I opted for something I knew was going to give me a boost of energy.

If I fancied a chocolate cake, I'd eat it, but I kept an extensive food diary of how it made my body feel. And the answer? Well, I was sitting on the loo about twelve hours later. Now I find swaps for the things I love that love my body too. You don't have to give up everything you love, but always be aware and in tune with your body and how what you put in is making it feel.

If you feel sluggish, with little energy, *you probably already know your answer.*

Our bodies are amazing things, they come in all shapes and sizes. They are hard-working machines, they exude beauty and we have the ultimate control of maintaining them and treating them well.

4. If in doubt, be kind

Kindness is so underrated and I try to bring it into every situation, regardless of how upset I am, how frustrated I can be or how angry or offended I am.

Take, for example, when I receive criticism on my YouTube channel or a certain Instagram post. Many people might argue that I should expect this kind of backlash because I'm actively putting my life online and up for discussion with those watching. I totally understand that.

But when somebody takes time out of their day to leave negativity, I question what could be going on in their day to feel the need to do this. Because a happy, self-fulfilled, driven and positive person doesn't leave negativity in someone else's life. If it's constructive and is written in a way that is trying to provide helpful support, then that's totally different. If someone critiques my lighting and says a video is too bright, that's not negativity. That's feedback and I'm all for improving my work.

I can take the comment how I want to (usually, I'll agree), but my understanding of negativity is where someone has taken the time to be hurtful, nasty, unhelpful and unkind to you. A message that isn't constructive at all, but that exudes an air of bitterness. Because, as I said, a happy, fulfilled person doesn't feel the need to be nasty about another person's life.

If I ever do receive these type of comments – and it happens, quite often – then my instinct is to react with kindness because I think it's the only helpful way you can deal with an unhappy person who invites and projects negativity onto someone who doesn't deserve it.

I think it's important to always try to be kind - even if it's difficult - because if we react with the same negativity, it only embroils you into the rabbit hole of negativity too.

We also never know what the commenter is going through in their day-to-day life. And although nothing excuses bad behaviour, I don't want to cause them more upset. I would hate to be the protagonist in making someone's day worse.

So if they throw a nasty comment my way, I'll wish them a good day or say that I'm sorry they're not having a great day but that I'm there to chat if they need to.

You might be completely ignored or a barrage of insults might be hurled back, or they might stop, apologise and realise that you're human too and don't deserve what has been thrown at you.

It says a lot about a person, the way they react, but you cannot control their reaction. You can only control your actions and if in doubt, *be kind.*

Kindness always wins. Nice always trumps nasty.

5. You're carving your own path

It's important not to compare your chapter 2, to someone else's chapter 20. Everyone is at a different stage in their life, which isn't necessarily relative to age or experience. We all experience different things, we have different things to offer.

Nobody else in this world is like you. Even if you have an identical twin, there's still something you offer that's different to them.

You are YOU and you're carving your own path. Your story is so different and so unique, it's not worth comparing it to anyone else's.

It doesn't gain anything and as the saying goes 'comparison is the thief of joy', so don't deprive yourself of happiness because you're putting your story and another's side by side.

Plus, much of the time, we're comparing our reality to another person's highlights reel, so it's completely incomparable anyway.

Don't worry about what others are doing, how fast they're progressing and what their goals are.

The most beautiful things in nature aren't concerned with whether something is blooming greater than they are, they just bloom the best they can. Similarly, everything and everyone is a genius, but if you judged a fish by its ability to climb a tree, it would go through life thinking it was stupid. We're all carving our own path.

Some people are better at different things, but that doesn't define **YOU**. You'll find your thing, just trust and put faith in the journey.

Honour your pace and admire others journey's without questioning your own.

6. Be content that life is a journey, not a destination

This is probably one of my favourite and most important rules of all, because we're all guilty of being caught up in the 'race' – reaching for our goals, working hard, achieving but striving for the next thing.

I am constantly asking myself, *'What's next?'* and while this is arguably proof of quite how driven I am, it's key that I enjoy, savour and praise the moment rather than constantly looking forward to what's ahead of me.

Because if I continue in this way, I'm going to miss the journey.

If I keep pushing for the next goal without appreciating the journey to it, I'm going to feel pretty unfulfilled by the time I reach those goals. *It's a catch 22.*

The joy is not found in finishing an activity, but doing it.

The irony and paradox of the human condition is that we are so focused with reaching 'THE pinnacle point' on our journey, a goal, or some happiness, that we seem to forget it's the journey itself where life happens.

It's the journey we'll cherish when we're old, not the completion of a momentary goal.

It's definitely worth having goals, but we should be contented in the fact that life isn't a one-dimensional destination.

Some of the most beautiful chapters in our lives won't have a title until much later.

You never know what pages the surprises, twists and love will feature on until you start reading the book.

And it's the art of devouring of the pages of the book, not the feeling of completion, that is most enjoyable.

"Enjoy, embrace and encourage the vivid dance of life!"

7. You don't always have to be tough

When I was younger, I thought I had to be tough in order to succeed. I thought I had to restrict my emotions, stay strong and be there for everyone else. Particularly with my mum, who I always had an innate urge to protect, look after and be emotionally robust for.

I thought that by wearing armour, I was protecting myself and earning the respect of others.

But in reality, your emotions are not a weakness, they are a strength. It takes a strong person to express how they feel, to let their emotions run wild and go with their gut instinct.

I will openly admit that I'm a very sensitive person. I now wear my heart on my sleeve and *sometimes*, this can be at my own detriment, but I'm not ashamed of it. I'm open, I'm aware and in tune with my own needs. When others show emotion it makes me feel connected not uncomfortable. I show that I care and I give myself permission to feel.

Feeling is one of our key instincts, it's what makes us human.

The human brain is insanely incredible. We have coping and defence mechanisms, we can put ourselves into fight or flight mode and build up our own adrenaline in preparation for something. We allow ourselves to feel pain, loss, grief, relief, drive, disappointment and happiness.

Feeling is powerful and by allowing ourselves to feel, we also acknowledge that all emotions are temporary. Happiness is not a constant state of mind but an emotion, and we need all that goes with happiness (sadness, frustration, anger) in order to appreciate the glory of being able to bask in happiness.

You don't always have to be tough *because there is merit in feeling and power in emotions.*

8. Embrace the shades of grey

And nope, don't worry – I'm NOT talking about that book. But life isn't black and white, like we imagine it is when we're a child. Life isn't about deciphering who is the '*good guy*' and who is a '*bad guy*'. But that's how we made sense of things when we were young, so we carry it with us through life too.

Just because someone makes a mistake, it doesn't mean they're inherently bad. I recently watched a film called *A Monster Calls*, which has a wonderful premise and is also incredibly heart wrenching. It brought home this very important life lesson through a series of stories, as told by the monster.

Sometimes good people make bad choices, it doesn't mean they are bad, it means they are human.

Take our parents, for example. When we're young we put them on a pedestal, we believe they can do no wrong. We look up to them, and rightly so. I know my parents are both incredible people, but I also know they've made mistakes and I would never judge them for that. Equally, I would expect them to guide me in the right direction, but also let me make my own mistakes and not say, '*I told you so,*' but just be there to pick me up.

Real life, the exciting things in life, the scary things in life – they all happen within the shades of grey. *So embrace them!*

9. Everything is subject to change

And change is good.

I suppose I've been quite lucky in the sense I had to get used to change from a young age.

My parents divorced when I was 8 years old, and from then onwards, we moved house every couple of years until we settled around aged 13-14.

So I've never really been sentimental about a family home nor have I tied sentimental value to certain objects or situations.

Change has been a big part of my life and I've always just got on with it.

However, I suppose unwelcome changes can still shock you and still permeate your life and it's more so about how you deal with them, then what they are.

And when you self-reflect, sometimes you realise that change is needed in order to progress.

As Einstein once said: "*Insanity is doing the same thing over and over and over and expecting a different result.*"

And so it might be that you're worried about the upheaval of quitting your job, or coming out of a negative relationship or friendship or making sacrifices for a longer-term goal.

But *"When the caterpillar thought the world was over, it became a butterfly."*

Perhaps a slightly cringeworthy quote but an important one at that.

In the beginning, change is hard, it's messy, it's emotional, but a year down the line, you'll forget who you were before. We're always growing as a person, and to grow, to change and to overcome, is to live. ·

Change is the only constant we can rely on in life, so we have to embrace it, love it and let it *encourage us to cherish moments before they become memories.*

"When the caterpillar thought the world was over, it became a butterfly."

Thank you for reading!

Love, Scarlett x

Resources

FOR RECIPES:

Deliciously Ella

Little Blog of Vegan

Niomi Smart

Madeleine Shaw

BOOKS I RECOMMEND:

The Life-Changing Magic of Not Giving a F**k - Sarah Knight

The Anxiety Solution: A Quieter Mind, a Calmer You - Chloe Brotheridge

The Complete Low Fodmap Solution - Dr Sue Shepherd

The Chimp Paradox: The Mind Management Programme to Help You Achieve Success, Confidence and Happiness - Professor Steve Peters

Mind Over Mood, Second Edition: Change How You Feel by Changing the Way You Think - Christine A. Padesky

Get The Glow: Delicious and Easy Recipes That Will Nourish You from the Inside Out - Madeleine Shaw

Eat.Nourish.Glow - Amelia Freer

ONLINE RESOURCES

Healthline

The IBS Network

IBS Support Groups on Facebook (the one I've created is called IBS Support Group by Scarlett London – creative name, I know)

NHS Guidance

Doctor's Kitchen Podcasts

Food
& Symptom Diary

Day	Breakfast	Lunch	Dinner	Snacks	Fluids & Activity	Symptoms & Comments
MONDAY: EXAMPLE...	2 WEETABIX WITH 1/2 CUP OF MILK, 1 TSP OF SUGAR	FILLED ROLL & APPLE	BEEF STIR FRY, 1/2 CUP RICE AND HALF PLATE OF VEGETABLES	YOGHURT, 2 X WATER CRACKERS, 2 X BISCUITS	WATER: ALCOHOL: EXERCISE:	SOME BLOATING BY 8PM, LOOSE MOTIONS X2, SETTLES BY BEDTIME
TUESDAY					WATER: ALCOHOL: EXERCISE:	
WEDNESDAY					WATER: ALCOHOL: EXERCISE:	

Day	Breakfast	Lunch	Dinner	Snacks	Fluids & Activity	Symptoms & Comments
THURSDAY					WATER: ALCOHOL: EXERCISE:	
FRIDAY					WATER: ALCOHOL: EXERCISE:	
SATURDAY					WATER: ALCOHOL: EXERCISE:	
SUNDAY					WATER: ALCOHOL: EXERCISE:	

53033852R00197

Made in the USA
San Bernardino, CA
11 September 2019